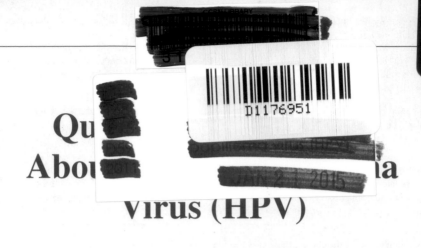

Qu
Abou
Virus (HPV)

Don S. Dizon, MD, FACP

Program in Women's Oncology
Women & Infants Hospital of Rhode Island
The Warren Alpert Medical School of Brown University
Providence, RI

Michael L. Krychman, MD

Medical Director of Sexual Medicine, Hoag Memorial Hospital Presbyterian
Executive Director of the Southern California Center for Sexual Health
and Survivorship Medicine
Associate Clinical Professor, University of Southern California
AASECT Certified Sexual Counselor

JONES AND BARTLETT PUBLISHERS
Sudbury, Massachusetts
BOSTON   TORONTO   LONDON   SINGAPORE

World Headquarters

Jones and Bartlett Publishers
40 Tall Pine Drive
Sudbury, MA 01776
978-443-5000
info@jbpub.com
www.jbpub.com

Jones and Bartlett Publishers
Canada
6339 Ormindale Way
Mississauga, Ontario L5V 1J2
Canada

Jones and Bartlett Publishers
International
Barb House, Barb Mews
London W6 7PA
United Kingdom

Jones and Bartlett's books and products are available through most bookstores and online book-sellers. To contact Jones and Bartlett Publishers directly, call 800-832-0034, fax 978-443-8000, or visit our website, www.jbpub.com.

The authors, editor, and publisher have made every effort to provide accurate information. However, they are not responsible for errors, omissions, or for any outcomes related to the use of the contents of this book and take no responsibility for the use of the products and procedures described. Treatments and side effects described in this book may not be applicable to all people; likewise, some people may require a dose or experience a side effect that is not described herein. Drugs and medical devices are discussed that may have limited availability controlled by the Food and Drug Administration (FDA) for use only in a research study or clinical trial. Research, clinical practice, and government regulations often change the accepted standard in this field. When consideration is being given to use of any drug in the clinical setting, the healthcare provider or reader is responsible for determining FDA status of the drug, reading the package insert, and reviewing prescribing information for the most up-to-date recommendations on dose, precautions, and contraindications, and determining the appropriate usage for the product. This is especially important in the case of drugs that are new or seldom used.

Production Credits

Executive Publisher: Christopher Davis
Editorial Assistant: Sara Cameron
Associate Production Editor: Leah Corrigan
Senior Marketing Manager: Barb Bartoszek
Manufacturing and Inventory Supervisor:
    Amy Bacus
Composition: Glyph International

Cover Design: Carolyn Downer
Cover Images: © Jason Stitt/
    ShutterStock, Inc., © Monkey Business
    Images/Dreamstime.com
Printing and Binding: Malloy, Inc.
Cover Printing: Malloy, Inc.

Library of Congress Cataloging-in-Publication Data
Dizon, Don S.
    Questions & answers about human papilloma virus (HPV) / Don S. Dizon,
Michael L. Krychman.
        p. cm.
    Includes index.
    ISBN 978-0-7637-8162-0 (alk. paper)
    1. Papillomavirus diseases—Miscellanea. 2.
Papillomaviruses—Miscellanea. 3. Generative
organs—Infections—Miscellanea. I. Krychman, Michael L. II. Title. III.
Title: Questions and answers about human papilloma virus (HPV).
    RC168.P15D59 2011
    616.9'11—dc22
                                            2009052706

6048

Printed in the United States of America
14 13 12 11 10   10 9 8 7 6 5 4 3 2 1

As always, I want to thank my publisher, Chris Davis, and friends at Jones and Bartlett for the opportunity to collaborate with Michael on this book. This book is dedicated to my spouse, Henry, and our children, Isabelle, Harrison, and Sophia, who are my support and inspiration for the work I do. I also want to dedicate it to the best parents in the world, Millionita and Modesto Dizon, who gave me every opportunity in the world to succeed from our little island in the South Pacific. This is also for my sisters, Michelle, Maerica, Precy, and Marie; their husbands, Mel, Ben, and Ed; and my niece and nephew, Stella and Jude. Lastly, I want to dedicate this to the people on my home island of Guam. Although far away, it will always be home to me.

—Don S. Dizon, MD, FACP

To my healthcare team, I thank you for your support. For my parents, the Franconis and Krychmans—a special thank you for the unconditional encouragement during my career. To my co-author Don Dizon, I am thankful for our friendship and am honored to have you as an esteemed colleague in oncology and sexual medicine. To my good friend and colleague, Susan, who has always encouraged me— your friendship has been a source of inspiration. For Bryanna, I hope all this talk about HPV has not completely scared you. Thank you to Chris Davis and the Jones and Bartlett team for their hard work and dedication.

And last but not least, for all the men and women, young and old, married, single, divorced, heterosexual and homosexual, who are desperate for education about HPV, its effects, and its treatment. I do hope this book can help ease the suffering and distress.

—Michael L. Krychman, MD

Contents

Contents

Viruses have always plagued humans and none in more ways than the human papilloma viruses. These can cause all sorts of human diseases from the "annoying," like warts, to the very serious, like cancer. They affect both men and women and, as such, can be considered "equal opportunity" infections.

As an oncologist I have been fascinated by the idea that an infection can cause cancer. This concept is best illustrated through the actions of the human papilloma virus, or HPV. It infects both men and women and is associated with cancers of the head and neck, penis, cervix, anal canal, vagina, and vulva. In addition, infections from HPV can cause other illnesses which are a significant source of human suffering, like warts on the face, feet, and even the genitals.

That one virus can cause all of this damage may seem astounding—but it is important to understand that HPV is not *one* virus, but rather, it is a family of multiple viruses, with varying propensities towards some diseases but not others. Hence, some HPV types can place one at an increased risk of cervical cancer, but another type altogether can be responsible for nothing more serious than warts. Because of the various ways infection with HPV can manifest, it remains one of the most interesting to study and learn about. This book aims to give the general reader an introduction to HPV, the diseases it is associated with, and more importantly, emphasizes modes of protection, and now, prevention.

Our hope is to stimulate the public into forging a more informed alliance with healthcare professionals to create a rational and evidence-based approach into ways to control HPV infection. We now have an opportunity to reduce the incidence of diseases associated with HPV—possible today with the FDA approval of HPV vaccines against certain strains. These first strides will hopefully usher in a new era in protection, one that our children and their children will benefit from.

Don S. Dizon, MD, FACP and Michael L. Krychman, MD

PART ONE

The Basics

What is a virus?

How do viruses make humans sick once
they enter the body?

How do humans fight off viruses?

More . . .

1. What is a virus?

A *virus* is an infectious agent that requires a host cell in order to multiply. Outside of the host, it is generally asleep (or *inert*). However, when it comes into contact with a human cell that it can infect, it inserts its genetic material (DNA or RNA) into its host and can take over the host cell's function. It then uses the cell's machinery to duplicate and multiply the virus. As a result, the host cell spits out more viruses, killing the host cell and leading to the release of more viruses. In general, viruses have three parts: genes; a protective coat that surrounds the genes, usually made of proteins; and outside of the host cell, an **envelope**—a membrane that surrounds the virus so it can live. Viruses have many different sizes and shapes, but they are always very small—nearly 1/100th the size of bacteria. When one speaks of one virus particle, it is called a virion; the pleural of virion is viruses. The word "virus" is actually Latin, which translates to "poison."

Viruses do not only infect human beings. Every plant, animal, and bacteria can become infected with a virus. In addition, not all viruses cause human diseases; some can multiply but cause no signs of illness. However, the viruses of concern impact humans by their ability to cause disability and even death. Throughout history, many viruses have caused disease for humans. Some of these diseases may be serious, while others are not severe.

2. How many viruses are there? Are there different kinds of virus?

There are more than 5000 viruses that scientists have been able to identify and fully describe in the medical literature. They are not all the same and are classified based on what characteristics the viruses have in common,

Envelope

A membrane that surrounds a virus so it can live.

There are more than 5000 viruses that scientists have been able to identify and fully describe in the medical literature.

called a **taxonomy**. In the current taxonomy, there are five virus orders (or *-virales* in Latin): Caudovirales, Herpesvirales, Mononegavirales, Nidovirales, and Picornavirales. However, only half of the named viruses have been described completely enough to make classifying them possible, so this is a work in continual progress and may be changed from time to time.

Beyond order, viruses are also classified by how they make copies of themselves, or replicate. In order to do this, their genetic material (or genome) must be made into **messenger RNA (mRNA)**, which is the blueprint by which proteins are produced. These proteins will eventually make the parts required to produce a new copy of the virus. Viruses may be DNA-based or RNA-based; comprised of one strand of genetic material, or have two strands; or require a special protein to manufacture proteins from their genetic material. This is highlighted in **Figure 1**. As you can see, the process of classification is highly complex and points to the significant genetic differences between the known viruses.

Taxonomy

Classification system based on the characteristics viruses have in common.

Messenger RNA (mRNA)

The blueprint by which proteins are produced.

The Basics

Figure 1   Genetic Make-up of a Virus.

3

3. What does a virus look like?

Viruses are as different from each other as people are. They are incredibly small—even smaller than bacteria. It is approximated that they are less than 300 nanometers in size, or less than one trillionth of an inch! Viruses are so small that they cannot even be seen by a light microscope. Instead, a specialized microscope called an electron microscope is often needed to see them.

4. Do viruses have a common structure?

Capsid

A shell that surrounds the virus, generally made up of proteins.

Genome

The complete genetic information of a virus or other organism.

Yes, all viruses generally have the same elements. They have a shell, called a **capsid**, that gives them protection and is encoded in their genes, which are contained in the genome. The **genome** is where the genetic material is housed, and, as noted in Question 2, it can be DNA- or RNA-based, single- or double-stranded, with a -sense (meaning that the DNA can be translated as-is into RNA and go on to construct proteins) or an antisense strand (meaning it is the complementary strand) present, and it can have its own protein to help it reproduce (the reverse transcriptase).

5. Do viruses infect humans in the same way?

No, not all viruses infect humans the same way. Think of the common cold—this illness is spread by a virus when infected people cough on each other or come in close contact. The virus then travels through the air and can infect those people who are nearby.

Hepatitis, a disease that can affect the liver, is also spread by a virus, but it is spread by infected people by contact with blood—usually when a non-infected person receives a blood transfusion from someone who is infected or through sharing of needles used to inject drugs (intravenous or IV drugs). Hepatitis also can be transmitted when a person comes in contact with other blood products. Viruses also can infect human beings by going through an intermediary, such as an insect. The mosquito is a common source of virus spread, and insects that generally carry infections from animals to humans are often termed **vectors**.

Other viruses, such as human Papilloma virus (HPV), is spread through sexual contact. HPV may be transmitted through direct contact (oral to genital, oral to oral, skin to skin), although it is typically transmitted through the skin-to-skin route. The virus also may spread by touching something that has been contaminated with HPV and then touching the skin, but it is unknown if, or how often, this occurs. Another method of transmission occurs when a person infects him- or herself, called **auto inoculation**, although this is thought to be a rare method of transmission. Transmission most often occurs by person-to-person contact. However, it is unlikely that HPV transmission can occur when the levels of the virus in the body are low or undetectable.

Vectors
Insects that generally carry infections from animals to humans.

Auto inoculation
Method of virus transmission that occurs when a person infects him- or herself.

6. How do viruses make humans sick once they enter the body?

Once viruses infect a human cell, they go from an "off" position to an "on" position. They essentially release their own *genome*, or genetic make-up, into the cell, where the genome then inserts into the cell's DNA. Once there, the viruses take over the cell's machinery and make it the primary aim to make more viruses. Eventually the cell gets overwhelmed with virus particles and dies. In the process of dying, it also releases all the viral particles that have been made, thus speeding the spread of viral infections.

7. How do humans fight off viruses?

The human immune system is our defense against virus infections. Infected cells can indicate they are infected by attaching a piece of viral protein onto their surfaces. Once this "flag" is raised, fighter immune cells, called **T-cells**, are activated, recognize the viral flag as a non-human protein product, and produce specific T-cells against the virus. These "killer" T-cells then multiply or divide, seek out, and destroy the infected cells. As effective as this process is, it only works if the T-cells are working properly and the virus is in a place where T-cells can reach. Some viruses spread through the nervous system; they can evade the immune system. Other viruses infect human cells, insert their genes into human DNA, but then do nothing. These viruses remain asleep and do not kill cells, in which case they are **dormant**, or inactive.

T-cells

Immune cells that fight against viruses.

Dormant

Inactive. Dormant viruses do not kill host cells.

PART TWO

Basics About HPV

What is HPV?

Who can get HPV?

What kind of diseases are caused by HPV?

More . . .

8. What is HPV?

HPV stands for **human papilloma virus**. It is a member of the family Papillomaviridae. Within this classification system, it is a member of Group I; it is a double-stranded DNA virus. Interestingly, papilloma virus was discovered in 1935 when the scientist Francis Rous showed it could cause a type of skin cancer when he infected rabbits with it. This was the first demonstration that viruses could cause cancer in mammals.

To date, more than 100 human papilloma viruses (HPVs) have been identified.

Papilloma viruses are very diverse, and nearly all mammals and birds can get infected by them. To date, more than 100 human papilloma viruses (HPVs) have been identified.

HPV infects both skin and mucus membranes, and not all of them behave the same way. Some cause serious diseases, while others are associated with less severe or benign diseases. HPV infections have been associated with cancer; the viruses have caused more than 500,000 cases of cancer worldwide, representing 5% of all cancers that are diagnosed each year.

Carol says:

Until the recent introduction of the HPV vaccine, many weren't aware that HPV isn't a single virus, but a group of strains. For example, just as dogs have different breeds, HPV has 100+ different strains. Different strains of HPV can cause different infections, some are annoying, and some are more serious.

Simply described, HPV infections are considered either low- or high-risk for a person's health. Low-risk types cause genital warts (EGW), and some changes in cells of the cervix and vulva. High-risk types of infection lead to pre-cancerous changes in or cancer of the cervix and vulva.

9. Who can get HPV?

Anyone sexually active (having vaginal, anal, or oral intercourse) is at risk for genital infection from HPV. Men and women are at equal risk of infection, and it is estimated that three out of every four people will get an HPV infection during their lifetime. Because HPV is spread though direct contact, people are infected at young ages. Once we become sexually active, though, the risk of becoming infected increases, and the more partners someone has, the more likely he or she is to get the infection. It is important to know that as we age we are not "out of the woods;" older people can remain infected with HPV and in this way, can still transmit it to others.

Beyond sexual transmission, the routes of HPV transmission are not entirely clear. In fact, the risk of nonsexual transmission of these viruses is controversial. Some studies have detected HPV in the fingernails, raising the possibility that HPV can be passed on by simple hand-to-hand contact. However, while HPV has been *detected* in the hands, there is *no definitive medical proof* that it can be transmitted this way. There is some evidence to suggest that HPV can be transmitted from mother to child (**vertical transmission**), and HPV infection at infancy can lead to a rare condition where warts occur in the respiratory tract (see Question 12). Not much is known about oral transmission of HPV, nor about how HPV creates an infection in the oral cavity. It is known that HPV infection of the oral cavity can result in cancer of the oral cavity or other areas of the head and neck. However, it is generally thought that oral–genital contact is the predominant form of transmission of HPV into the oral cavity.

Vertical transmission

Passing of a virus from mother to child.

10. How is HPV spread?

When someone is exposed to HPV, the virus usually enters through microscopic tears in the skin. After entering the skin, it loses its shell (or capsid), allowing its genetic material (DNA) to enter into the human host cell's nucleus, where it lives separately from the host cell's DNA. The viral DNA can then multiply within the human cell. This initial infection occurs quite commonly. In one study from Seattle, 20% of women entering college who participated in HPV screening were already HPV DNA-positive at the beginning of the study. In the first two years of medical follow-up, the percentage increased to 39%, with the most common viral infections involving HPV 16 and 18 (two different subtypes of the HPV virus). By the end of the six-year study, 80% of the women were HPV DNA-positive.

As the infection persists, infected cells mature and become a part of the skin structure as the virus starts making copies of itself independently of the infected cell. Once HPV starts to replicate, it also gets ready to leave the infected cell by making proteins that will coat it in a *capsid*. Once the infected cells reach the most outer layer of the skin, the virus daughters repackage themselves and leave. When the HPV begins leaving, the cell experiences changes that are profoundly abnormal; it is these cells that can be picked up on a Pap smear as proof of an HPV infection.

Unlike other viruses that are sexually transmitted, such as human immunodeficieny virus (HIV), HPV is not transmitted through semen or other bodily fluids. It is also important to know that most women who become infected do not remain so; in the vast majority of women, the infection is transient and will be cleared by her immune system. In fact, the proportion of women with persistent infections ranges from less than 1% to about 20%.

Carol says:

It should be a simple deduction—HPV is in the group of STD's, so sexual transmission is how it's spread. But, there are times when patients find out they have an HPV infection and haven't been sexually active for weeks. How does this happen?

Friction in genital skin to skin contact is the surprising answer for many. This is one aspect that makes it easy to assume that if one partner is infected, the other will be, too. HPV operates on its own set of rules and travels from person to person without any warning signs. If HPV could speak, "maybe" would be its favorite word. Maybe it's going to appear in a new host person, or maybe not. Maybe it will show symptoms, or maybe not. Maybe if it's present the symptoms will go away on their own, or maybe not. It's ambiguous, opportunistic, and seems to act on a whim. And it's unknown how long any of the "maybe" process takes.

So, what is clear about HPV is that there are no clear-cut answers to many aspects of how it spreads.

11. Are there any statistics that state how many people are infected?

HPV infection is the most common genital infection in the United States. Estimates place the number of people infected with HPV within the United States at 20 million people, with approximately half of those aged 15 to 25 years. By age 50, it is expected that up to 80% of sexually active women are infected with HPV. Despite this, most people infected with HPV have no symptoms and thus are unaware they are infected.

Worldwide, HPV DNA-positivity is highest among women under 20, in whom the rates are almost three times higher than in women in their 40s and 50s.

Worldwide, HPV DNA-positivity is highest among women under 20, in whom the rates are almost three times higher than in women in their 40s and 50s. This likely is more reflective of when women get infected (at an early age), and the majority of women clear the infection by the time they reach their 50s. A second increase in the rate of HPV positivity occurs in women in their 60s. While the reason for this is not entirely clear, it may reflect that HPV, which was in essence "asleep" during most of a woman's life, starts to replicate later in life.

12. What kinds of diseases are caused by HPV?

For women, HPV is the single most important biologic risk factor for developing genital warts and both pre-cancerous and cancerous lesions of the genital track, including those involving the cervix, vulva, vagina, and anal canal. In men, HPV is a major risk factor for the development of both anus and penile cancers.

The risk of cervical cancer is intimately tied to the type of HPV infection present. For example, there is more than a 400-fold increased risk of cervical cancer if a girl or woman has HPV 16, compared with those not infected with HPV-16. To place it in proper perspective, such a risk factor is far higher than that of lung cancer for smokers (where it is 8-fold higher) or breast cancer for women on hormone replacement therapy (where it is about 1.3-fold higher).

Beyond the genital area, HPV is associated with increased risk of cancers involving the head and neck, particularly a squamous cell cancer of the oropharynx. One study showed that overall, 26% of tumors were positive for HPV. Some members of the HPV family can also cause body warts. Those in the genital area are called condyloma accuminata or **venereal warts**. Those on the soles of one's foot are called **plantar warts**; those on the face are called **flat warts**. Warts can also form anywhere in the respiratory tract, from the larynx into the lungs. This very rare condition in the lungs is known as *respiratory Papillomatosis* and can cause trouble breathing, which in some cases can be fatal; 1–3% of people with it usually die from it. The disease is usually acquired during birth and may require surgery to manage it. Another HPV disease of the skin is called *epidermodysplasia verruciformis*, where scaly patches form on the skin, particularly on the hands and feet; it can be both non-cancerous and cancerous. We will touch on the more serious diseases associated with HPV in greater detail later.

Carol says:

Basically, a skin area exposed to an area of infected skin can result in an infection. In women, the vulva, vagina, and cervix are HPV infection targets. One way to think about it is imagining the diseases on a stairway with steps that go up to a landing, and then down again.

In this picture, the lowest step of HPV infection is genital warts, caused by one group of the virus strains.

A different group of strains cause pre-cancer conditions are on the next step: CIN in the cervix, VIN of the vulva, and VAIN in the vagina. The cervix and vulva have different grades of pre-cancer. Because the mention of cancer can block hearing and stop learning, it's important to understand that that pre-cancer is not cancer and does not necessarily become cancer. Terms that describe cervical changes from low to high are: "ASCUS" (Atypical Squamous Cells of Undetermined Significance), "LSIL" (Low-grade Intraepithelial Lesion) = "CIN 1" (Cervical Intraepithelial

Venereal warts
Body warts in the genital area.

Plantar warts
Warts on the soles of the foot.

Flat warts
Warts on the face.

Basics About HPV

Neoplasia-1) are in this group. In the vulva, the lowest grade is VIN-1 (Vulvar Intraepithelia Neoplasia-1).

On the next step up, more of the region's tissue is occupied by abnormal cells. In the cervix, "HSIL" (High-grade Squamous Intraepithelial Lesion) = the CIN 2 or 3. In the vulva, it's VIN 2 or 3. In the vagina, VAIN (Vaginal Intraepithelia Neoplasia) is not graded.

Cervical, vulvar, or vaginal cancer is on the top step. CIN 3 and VIN 3 that are carcinoma in situ (cancer in place) are in this group as well. Vaginal cancer is a rare type of cancer.

Just as the steps go up, they can also go down before reaching the next higher step. Regular exams and follow-up help diseases move in a downward direction long before the top step is reached on this stairway.

13. What do we know specifically about how HPV works?

The virus infects skin cells, called keratinocytes, and takes over the replication process of these cells to multiply. Once the virus is present, a person can infect others. The high-risk HPV types such as HPV 16 and 18 encode early proteins known as E6 and E7, which promote tumors to grow and become malignant/cancerous; hence, they are known as *oncogenes*. These proteins work by blocking genes that suppress tumors from developing or growing. One of the proteins that these oncogenes blocks is known as p53. The p53 protein is part of an important pathway for getting rid of cells whose DNA has been damaged. Once the pathway is activated, it leads the cell to a natural death, or apoptosis. The end result is that when p53 is blocked, which in the case of HPV is due to the action of E6 and E7, cells are saved from dying naturally, a process called immortalization.

14. How are HPV viruses described?

Because there are many strains of HPV, they are often classified based on whether they are a low- or high-risk factor for causing diseases, especially cancer.

High-Risk Types

HPV types include 16, 18, 31, 33, 35, 39, 45, 51, 52, 56, 58, 59, 68, 73, and 82. Of these, HPV 16 and 18 are the most common infections found to cause cancer. HPV 16 is associated with more than half of the cervical cancers worldwide, and HPV 18 is associated with up to an additional 12% of cases.

Low-Risk Types

The low-risk HPV types, including HPV subtypes, are 6, 11, 40, 42, 43, 44, 54, 61, 70, 72, 81, and CP6108. In women, these viruses are often associated with abnormal Pap smear changes and external genital warts. A summary of the various HPV types and the diseases they are associated with is given in **Table 1**.

> *HPV 16 is associated with more than half of the cervical cancers worldwide, and HPV 18 is associated with up to an additional 12% of cases.*

15. How can you test for HPV?

For women, the **Pap test** or Papanicolaou smear (**Pap smear**) enables your healthcare provider to test for changes in the cervix, which may be related to an infection with HPV. However, the Pap test will not tell you if cervical changes mean you have an HPV infection.

We know that cervical cancer arises from pre-cancer changes and that it takes an average of 10 years for cancer of the cervix to develop from a high-grade lesion (or cervical intraepithelial neoplasia [CIN]). That this process takes so long allows your doctors to check for suspicious changes before they have a chance to become cancerous. This is also known as screening, because by catching those changes at an early phase, we can stop the cancerous process from being allowed to continue.

Pap test

Test for women that enables a healthcare provider to test for changes in the cervix, which may be related to an infection with HPV.

Table 1   Summary of HPV Types and Associated Diseases

Human Disease	HPV Type
Warts	
Common warts (verrucae vulgaris)	1, 2, 4, 26, 2, 29, 41, 57, 65
Those involving the soles of the feet (plantar)	1, 2, 4, 63
Those of the face (flat)	3, 10, 27, 28, 38, 41, 49
Those of the genitals or anus (anogenital)	6, 11, 30, 42, 43, 44, 45, 51, 52, 54
Respiratory papillomatosis	6, 11
Cervical dysplasia	6, 11, 16, 18, 30, 31, 33, 34, 35, 39, 40, 42, 43, 44, 45, 51, 52, 53, 56, 57, 58, 59, 61, 62, 64, 66, 67, 68, 69
Cervical cancer	16, 18
Penile cancer	16, 18
Vulvar cancer	6, 11, 16, 18
Vaginal cancer	16
Anal cancer	16, 31, 32, 33
Oral cancer	16, 18
Epidermodysplasia verruciformis	
Benign	2, 3, 10, 12, 15, 19, 36, 47, 50
Malignant	5, 8, 9, 10, 14, 17, 20, 21, 22, 23, 24, 25, 37, 38

In the United States, the most common type of Pap smear is the liquid-based Pap test, Thin Prep.

The Pap test is done when a woman has a pelvic exam. While lying down on the exam table the doctor places a special instrument called a speculum into the vagina and opens it in order to see the cervix. Once visualized a spatula and/or brush is used to take cells from inside and around the cervix. These cells are placed on a glass slide for examination. In the United States, the most common type of Pap smear is the liquid-based Pap test, Thin Prep.

For men, genital HPV testing is done by visual inspection for warts. Beyond this, there is no FDA-approved test for HPV detection in men. Some specialists advocate using a dilute solution of acetic acid on the penile tissue coupled with high resolution glasses to further examine the penis and detect HPV lesions. The Centers for Disease Control (CDC) does not feel testing is indicated because HPV is not likely to affect men's health. However, HIV-positive men who have low immune cell counts (known as CD-4 counts) or immunocompromised men are more likely to get HPV-associated diseases, including penile and anal cancers. Statistics cite that gay and bisexual men are 17 times more likely to develop HPV-related diseases. For these "at-risk" men, anal Pap smears are advocated by some experts, though they are not endorsed by the CDC.

Men or women who are at high risk for anal cancer may be recommended to undergo an anal Pap smear screening as well. Abnormal cells on these screening tests may signal the need for further testings and investigations to rule out serious underlying diseases. We will touch on this later in the book.

There is also a specialized test that checks for HPV DNA, the genetic material of the virus itself. It can be indicated as a follow-up test if a Pap test returns with some types of abnormal results. The HPV DNA test can determine whether a high-risk type of HPV caused the abnormal Pap test. Women with a normal Pap test and no HPV infection have a very low risk for developing cervical cancer. However, those women with both an abnormal Pap test and a positive HPV test have a risk at 6% or greater for developing cervical cancer, so they warrant further investigation and follow-up. The HPV DNA test is currently FDA-approved as a screening test along with the Pap test in women over the age of 30. However, it does not substitute for regular Pap tests nor is it intended as a screen for women under age 30.

The American College of Obstetricians and Gynecologists recently updated their recommendations for cervical cytology screening as follows:

- Cervical cancer screening should begin at age 21 years regardless of sexual activity.
- Cytologic screening is recommended every 2 years for women ages 21 to 29.
- Women 30 years and older in a monogamous relationship with negative cytology and negative high-risk HPV test may have screening every 3 years.
- Women over 30 years with three consecutive negative Pap tests and no risk factors may be screened every 3 years.
- Screening should be more frequent in high-risk groups, including: women infected with the human immunodeficiency virus (HIV), immunocompromised women, women with a history of DES exposure in utero, and women previously treated for CIN 2, 3 or cervical cancer.

Reflex HPV testing
Screens for the presence or absence of high-risk HPV typology when a cell test from a Pap smear is abnormal.

Some providers use **reflex HPV testing**—when the cell test from the Pap smear is abnormal, the reflex test screens for the presence or absence of high-risk HPV typology.

Carol says:

Some people know their partners are positive for HPV, and then wonder if they have the virus, too. For them, finding out there is no screening test is disappointing and can cause more uncertainty and anxiety. In this case, emphasizing regular screening and practicing prevention puts some control back in the situation.

Until a screening test is available, regular gynecologic exams with pap test screenings are the best basic plan of action. Based on abnormal pap test results, further screen testing with a colposcopy can be used for further investigation.

PART THREE

HPV and Cervical Disease

What is cervical dysplasia?

How is cervical dysplasia diagnosed?

How is cervical dysplasia treated?

More . . .

16. What is cervical dysplasia?

Approximately 50 million women undergo a Pap test each year, of which 7% have some type of abnormality that requires an evaluation.

Cervical dysplasia describes changes in the cells of the cervix, seen only under a microscope, that are precancerous lesions. These lesions are far more common than cervical cancer. Approximately 50 million women undergo a Pap test each year, of which 7% have some type of abnormality that requires an evaluation. Low-grade lesions of the cervix are diagnosed in approximately 1 million women, while an additional half a million may have higher grade lesions that would require further evaluation. Many of the low-grade lesions so often resolve spontaneously that many healthcare providers will choose close follow-up or surveillance when the lesions are low grade—a repeat Pap smear often is recommended at a shorter interval than it would be typically. High-grade lesions prompt referral for further evaluation to rule out cancer and for definitive treatment.

Carol says:

A screening test may come back showing cervical dysplasia. But when someone hears those words, it can sound like a foreign language and scary. Understanding the terms and the meanings builds a good foundation and are basic to understanding implications of cervical dysplasia.

A very simple anatomy lesson is a good place to start. It's not uncommon for some to use the term "vagina" to refer to all of the female reproductive area. Pictures of the structures show the cervix is a structure like a donut-shaped "gate" located between the vagina below and the uterus above.

Learning how cervical cells grow is next. Dysplasia describes a process of abnormal cell growth. The more immature cells there are, the more abnormal the growth is of the cervical tissue. Sometimes the term "lesion" is also used to describe the damage of this process. Cervical dysplasia means that normal cervical cells are replaced with abnormal immature ones, which is the first step in moving towards a pre-cancerous state.

17. How is cervical dysplasia diagnosed?

Cervical dysplasia is suggested by an abnormal Pap test. As discussed in Question 15, a Pap test is performed by inserting a speculum into the vagina, which enables your doctor to see the cervix deep within the vaginal vault. Using a tiny spatula or swab, a sample of the cervical cells is obtained and then put on a glass slide and sent to the laboratory. Typically, the Pap test will evaluate for the presence of precancerous cervical lesions, although cervical cancer also can be identified. If the Pap test is abnormal, your doctor may require coloposcopy and subsequent biopsy, which is how dysplasia is definitively diagnosed. Coloposcopy is discussed in Question 19.

18. Are there different types of dysplasia?

Yes, there are different types of dysplastic lesions and the American Society for Colposcopy and Cervical Pathology (ASCCP) has a great brochure on this. For more information visit: http://www.asccp.org/patient_edu.shtml. The system used to classify dysplastic lesions is called the Bethesda Pap Test Classification System. General categories in the Bethesda system are "negative for intraepithelial lesion or malignancy," "epithelial cell abnormality," or "other." If an epithelial cell abnormality is found, it is described as a squamous cell or a glandular cell. Squamous epithelial findings are further characterized into atypical squamous cells of undetermined significance (ASC-US); cannot exclude high-grade squamous intraepithelial

The system used to classify dysplastic lesions is called the Bethesda Pap Test Classification System.

lesion (ASC-H); low-grade squamous intraepithelial lesion (LGSIL); high-grade squamous intraepithelial lesion (HG-SIL); or squamous cell carcinoma. Glandular epithelial findings include atypical glandular cells (AGC), endocervical adenocarcinoma in situ (AIS), or adenocarcinoma.

ASC-US is generally considered a noncancerous finding. Atypia in this context means that the pathologist has found evidence of "irritation," but not enough to make a diagnosis of dysplasia. Approximately 70% of ASC-US lesions will revert or return to normal without anything further required. Although 7% of this type of lesion may progress to a higher grade over the next 2 years, the risk of progression to invasive cancer is extremely low. If ASC-US is found, repeat Pap tests may be recommended at 4 or 6 months. If HPV is present with ASC-US, you also may need repeat Pap smears at differing intervals.

As noted, AGC refers to glandular atypical cells. These are often more concerning because between 20–50% of women with this diagnosis may have a more severe lesion present, which could progress into cancer if untreated. Therefore, further workup and testing may be indicated after AGC-US is found; usually this means a colposcopy, which would allow your doctor to sample the endocervical canal. Another test which may be required with an AGC smear is an endometrial biopsy. During this test, the provider places a special pipelle within the uterine cavity and takes a small sample of the endometrial lining; it is then sent to the pathologist for analysis. Even when the pathology is unclear, some onoclogists may recommend a more invasive procedure called a cone biopsy.

19. How is cervical dysplasia treated?

Cervical dysplasia is treated based on multiple factors. The first is the age of the patient. It has been shown that as women get older, the rates of persistence of HPV and precancerous change (dysplasia) of the cervix increase. In older women, especially those who have completed childbearing, treatment is more likely to include an active intervention such as surgery or freezing of the lesion. The second factor in treatment is the patient's desire for fertility. A decision to perform a procedure on the cervix of a woman who wishes to have babies in the future must take into account the impact a procedure may have on the cervix. On rare occasions, a surgery may make it more difficult for a woman to carry a pregnancy to term. The third factor is the severity of the abnormal cervical finding. In the lowest grades of dysplasia, low-grade cervical dysplasia (LGSIL), the abnormality has a much higher likelihood of going away on its own, especially in women who are not smokers and have no significant problems with their body's immune system. If the LGSIL persists and does not regress or go away, the healthcare provider may suggest treatment. As the severity of the abnormal cervical finding increases, the likelihood of the abnormality going away on its own decreases, so watchful waiting is not used as often.

A **colposcopy** exam is a method of more closely evaluating the cervix of a woman with an abnormal Pap test. A colposcopy in combination with a biopsy is considered the best way to see if there is a precancerous or cancerous change of the cervix. Basically, colposcopy is a magnified view of the cervix by using a machine called a colposcope, which is a high-powered magnifying glass. The exam is performed in a fashion

It has been shown that as women get older, the rates of persistence of HPV and precancerous change (dysplasia) of the cervix increase.

Colposcopy

A method of more closely evaluating a woman with an abnormal Pap test by using a high-powered microscope to view the cervix.

HPV and Cervical Disease

23

quite similar to obtaining a Pap test—with the patient lying on her back with feet in stirrups and an instrument called a speculum inserted into the vagina. The cervix is gently wiped clean with a large Q-tip, and then either a dilute acetic acid solution (vinegar) or a substance called Lugol's solution (iodine) is applied to the cervix. The healthcare provider then looks through the colposcope at the cervix. During the exam, the healthcare provider looks for two important findings. First, the provider needs to see the entire transformation zone of the cervix. The **transformation zone** (much like a border between two different surfaces) is the place where the glandular cells that line the inside of the cervix meet the smooth skin cells that line the outside of the cervix. It is at that border that cells undergo change (transform) from one type of cell to the other. Sometimes the healthcare provider will use a green light on the colposcope to better visualize some of the changes that can occur on the cervix. During their transformation, cells are open to damage by outside influences such as HPV. Because of this, the transformation zone is the area of the cervix that is most commonly the site of precancerous or cancerous change. By seeing the entire transformation zone, the provider can be certain that the examination is adequate to make a judgment about whether there are any abnormal areas. Sometimes a biopsy is needed, in which the healthcare provider will take a small portion of the abnormal cervical tissue and send it off for pathological analysis. After the biopsy, a solution of silver nitrate often is placed on the biopsy site to stop the bleeding.

Transformation zone

The place where the glandular cells that line the inside of the cervix meet the smooth skin cells that line the outside of the cervix.

PART FOUR

HPV and Genital Warts

What are external genital warts (EGW)?

How are warts treated?

Are there non-surgical therapies for wart treatment?

More . . .

20. What are external genital warts (EGW)?

In women, warts are generally located in the areas exposed to friction during sexual activity, such as the posterior forchette, and can be found on the vulva, perineum, vagina, cervix, urethra, mouth, and larynx.

The classic appearance of **external genital warts** is a raised, peaked cauliflower-like lesion. However, they can also be flat, rough or smooth. It is estimated that up to 500,000 to 1 million new cases of EGW occur in the United States each year, and about 1% of sexually active men and women have visible warts at any one time. In women, warts are generally located in the areas exposed to friction during sexual activity, such as the posterior forchette, and can be found on the vulva, perineum, vagina, cervix, urethra, mouth, and larynx. Women may note the presence of a mass when warts are present, and there is a possibility that they can become infected, causing tenderness, spotting, or a foul odor. In men, genital warts present as growths on the penis, testicles, groin, anus, or thighs, and generally do not cause pain. Warts may appear within weeks or months following infection. Genital warts also might be found in the scar of an incision or in the area where a previous wart has been removed.

These lesions are usually caused by HPV 6 or 11 infection, though other types also are associated with EGW. Infections with warts are benign and do not lead to cancer, although many women and men may be concerned about the idea of having a sexually transmitted disease. Some people also think there is a social stigma associated with warts, and for some it may be sexually devestating.

21. What are the indications for biopsy of an EGW?

A warty lesion may be surrounded by thickened ulcerated or discolored skin; may be raised, bleeding, or an abnormal color; or may be fixed or indurated. All these situations may warrant a biopsy of the lesion. Other indications for biopsy may include those warts that are not responsive to local therapy or those lesions in women who are high risk, such as women who are infected with HIV or are heavy smokers. Some healthcare practitioners advocate that all warts should be biopsied so you have a correct diagnosis. A wart may look different than a lesion of some other form, so having an excisional biospy may be helpful.

22. How are warts treated?

Treatment of warts depends on the wart size, number of warts, wart location, possibility of adverse effects, cost, and patient preference. Some lesions may need to be removed by surgery, although this is usually reserved for large lesions. **Cryotherapy**, or surgical freezing, laser treatment, or the loop electrosurgical excision procedure (LEEP) are other treatment options. Cryotherapy using liquid nitrogen is the preferred treatment for urethral warts. Treatment using this method can be repeated every two weeks provided there is progress in reducing the lesions. Healthcare providers do not use cryotherapy for warts within the vagina because the depth of penetration maybe difficult to control, and care must be taken to avoid penetration of the vagina mucosa. Laser ablation maybe be very helpful where the lesions are widespread and unresponsive to other therapies.

Cryotherapy
Surgical freezing of warts, usually using liquid nitrogen.

23. Are there non-surgical therapies for wart treatment?

There are several types of medical therapies that are divided into patient- or healthcare provider-applied medical treatments. You must consider cost, comfort, duration, and the time it will take to clear the warts when choosing a product. Podofilox 0.5% gel is an agent that can destroy warts. It can be applied twice daily for 3 consecutive days for 4 weeks. According to the medical label, the treated surface must not exceed 10 cm^2 and no more than 0.5 mL of the gel should be used each day. Side effects include local inflammation, such as itching or bleeding, headaches, and even skin ulceration. Recurrence has been reported in up to 38% of patients treated, and long-term remission varies from 30–60%.

Carol says:

Patients want to get rid of the warts as soon as possible, but the idea of minor surgery or "cutting" is scary. With a few warts, medical treatment and some non-surgical procedures may be tried. Regardless of the method, managing treatment expectations involves three areas of treatment: the type, its length, and the outcome.

The treatment type is based on several factors. Medicines are directly applied to the warts by the healthcare provider or patient. Cryotherapy, or freezing, may be used to destroy the warts from the inside out. Initial treatment can take several applications over 4–16 weeks.

It's certainly encouraging to see warts disappearing as the treatment progresses. But just when things seem back to normal, it's common for new ones to appear, requiring treatment again. This is when persistence is a virtue!

24. What is imiquimod cream?

Imiquimod 5% cream is a cell-mediated immune response modifier that is applied to a warty lesion 3 times a week, alternating nights for up to 16 weeks. The cream is rubbed well into the lesion and washed off 6 to 10 hours after the application. Most patients will develop local redness and fewer than 10% will complain of pain. This medication is class C during pregnancy. Complete clearance of warts occurs in 50.5% of patients. The effects of this medication are considered long term, thus, recurrence of warts tends to be very low.

25. What is podophyllin?

Podophyllin is an antimitotic agent that works by stopping cells from growing. It is available as a cream or resin and should be applied directly to the wart until it disappears, which may take 6 weeks or longer. Up to 80% of patients will have resolution of their warts; however, up to 65% of patients may have recurrence after the treatment is completed. The most common side effects are burning, redness, pain, itching, and swelling. Podophyllin should not be used during pregnancy because of the risk to the fetus. This agent sometimes can have serious systemic implications, and some experts recommend against its use in primary care settings.

Podophyllin
An antimitotic agent that works by stopping cells from growing.

26. What is sinecatechins?

Sinecatechins is a new treatment available for the treatment of genital warts. This treatment is a plant-derived drug extract of green tea leaves and a mixture of bioflavonoids, polyphenols, and antioxidants. The ointment is applied 3 times a day in a thin layer for up to 16 weeks. In published clinical trials, clearance rates were 54%. Many women and men have interest in this method because it is derived from green tea leaves and, for some, is felt to be a more natural form of therapy than other treatment options.

PART FIVE

HPV and Cervical Cancer

What exactly is cervical cancer?

How big of a problem is cervical cancer?

How is cervical cancer treated?

More . . .

27. What exactly is cervical cancer?

When cells become abnormal and grow beyond their normal origin to become invasive, they become cancer. **Cervical cancer** occurs when these abnormal cells begin in the cervix. The most common cancers in the cervix originate within the cervix, although it also is a rare site to which other cancers may spread. The more common types of cancer that can spread to the cervix are cancers of the uterus or other female pelvic organs. There are a variety of invasive cervical cancer types; they are defined by the type of cells seen under the microscope. This means that the best way to tell what kind of cervical cancer a woman has is to perform a biopsy. The most common type of invasive cervical cancer is squamous cell carcinoma. **Squamous cells** are the cells that make up the majority of the skin lining throughout the body, including the cervix. Squamous cell carcinomas account for approximately 75% of all cervical cancers. There is one subtype of squamous cell carcinomas that is less aggressive than the others— villoglandular carcinoma. This type of tumor tends to have a growth pattern that stays on the cervix and rarely involves the surrounding tissue. The second most common type of squamous cell carcinoma is **adenocarcinoma**, which indicates that the cancer arose within the glands of the cervix. The glandular lining of the cervix is on its inner part, next to the uterus. These glandular cells also can be found throughout the lining tissues of the body, such as the in the colon and breasts.

Adenocarcinomas account for approximately 20% of all cancers of the cervix. Squamous cell carcinomas and adenocarcinomas of the cervix are associated with HPV, and testing for the virus in cancer specimens shows that almost 100% are positive. Stage-for-stage,

Cervical cancer

Occurs when abnormal cells begin in the cervix and grow beyond their normal origin to become invasive.

The most common type of invasive cervical cancer is squamous cell carcinoma.

Squamous cells

The cells that make up the majority of the skin lining throughout the body, including the cervix.

Adenocarcinoma

The second most common type of squamous cell carcinoma; indicates that the cancer arose within the glands of the cervix.

these two types of cervical cancers have similar rates of survival. Other cell types, which combined make up approximately 5% of all cancers of the cervix, include neuroendocrine carcinoma, melanoma, carcinosarcoma, serous adenocarcinoma, adenosquamous carcinoma, and lymphoma. Neuroendocrine cancers of the cervix are very aggressive. Even if diagnosed in early stage, they have a strong tendency recur, which reduces survival rates. Women with this diagnosis tend to undergo more extensive therapy due to the aggressive nature of this type of cancer. Lymphomas need to be identified, as treatment for these types of cancer differ greatly from the more common abnormal cell types.

While cervical cancer is fairly uncommon in the United States, it is the second most common cause of cancer-related death in women worldwide and the leading cause of cancer-related death in many developing countries. It is estimated that each year, more than 450,000 cases are diagnosed, and more than 230,000 deaths are recorded. Because cervical cancer can be diagnosed in younger women, it also is the leading cause of years of life lost due to cancer among women in their most productive years (between age 25 years and 64 years).

28. How is cervical cancer diagnosed if it is suspected on a Pap smear?

If a Pap smear comes back suspicious for high grade dysplasia or invasive cancer, a better examination of the cervix is indicated; this is accomplished by colposcopy. A colposcopy exam is a method of more closely evaluating the cervix of a woman with an abnormal Pap test, and it allows a piece of the cervix to be removed, which is known as a biopsy. A colposcopy uses a machine called a colposcope, which is a high-powered magnifying glass. With the patient positioned on her back on the examining table with her feet in stirrups, a speculum is inserted into the vagina. The cervix is gently wiped clean with a large Q-tip, and then either a dilute acetic acid solution (vinegar) or a substance called Lugol's solution (iodine) is applied to the cervix. This will magnify abnormal changes on the cervix so that your healthcare provider can perform a biopsy of the area of concern.

29. How is a cone biopsy performed?

If the original biospy warrents further treatment, the surgeon may recommend a **cone biopsy**. This is the most common surgery in women with suspicious findings from a colposcopy. If a woman has an abnormal Pap test but the colposcopy is normal, the abnormal area might be further inside the cervix. Because it is difficult to see, a cone biopsy may be performed in this circumstance as well.

Cone biopsy

The most common surgery in women with suspicious findings from a colposcopy.

A cone biopsy can be performed with a scalpel, loop electrosurgical excision procedure (LEEP), or laser. A cold-knife cone biopsy is the process of removing cervical tissue with a scalpel. A laser cone biopsy uses a laser beam as the method of cutting. A LEEP cone biopsy uses electrical energy conducted through a wire loop to cut tissue. Regardless of the technique utilized, the goal of a cone biopsy is to obtain enough tissue from both the outside and inside of the cervix to help diagnose precancerous change of the cervix.

The goal of a cone biopsy is to obtain enough tissue from both the outside and inside of the cervix to help diagnose precancerous change of the cervix.

Risks of cone biopsy include risks associated with any anesthesia, although the length of the procedure is shorter than other common operations. Most surgeons would consider a cone biopsy to fall into the category of a minor surgical procedure. However, on rare occasions, patients may experience bleeding or have an infection after the surgery that requires antibiotics. The most common long-term side effect of concern for women is the impact that a cone biopsy will have on their ability to become pregnant or maintain a pregnancy. A single cone biopsy has not been shown to decrease a woman's ability to become pregnant, and it rarely predisposes a woman to pre-term labor or losing a pregnancy.

Sometimes, in women who have more than one cone biopsy, a stitch (or **cerclage**) is placed in the cervix after they have become pregnant to help strengthen the cervix for the remainder of the pregnancy. An transvaginal ultrasound can help to determine if a woman will need a cerclage. Due to the need for this type of evaluation, women with a history of a cone biopsy who become pregnant should see an obstetrician early in pregnancy. Sometimes a high-risk perinatal consultation may be necessary.

Cerclage
A stitch placed in the cervix after a woman has become pregnant to help strengthen the cervix for the remainder of the pregnancy.

30. Is cervical intraepithelial neoplasia (CIN) cancer?

No, **cervical intraepithelial neoplasia (CIN)** is not cancer. Cervical intraepithelial neoplasia is another term for cervical dysplasia and is used to describe the findings on a cervical biopsy. Basically, this means that the normally uniform layers of cells seen within the cervix are not present. Cervical intraepithelial neoplasia is classified based on the degree of dysplasia, divided into CIN-I (low grade), or CIN-II or CIN-III (high grade). CIN-III is also referred to as *carcinoma in-situ*. Of these, CIN-III correlates strongly with infection with high-risk HPV. Cervical intraepithelial neoplasia is not the same as invasive cervical cancer, but it does represent preinvasive cervical carcinoma. High-grade CIN (CIN-II and CIN-III), however, requires excision of the affected area, which can be done using

Cervical intraepithelial neoplasia
Another term for cervical dysplasia and is used to describe the findings on a cervical biopsy.

multiple different techniques such as ablation or hysterectomy. High-risk cervical changes often progress to cervical cancer and should not be ignored.

31. How big of a problem is cervical cancer?

Invasive cervical cancer is not common in women within the United States where each year, approximately 11,000 women are diagnosed. Unfortunately, the worldwide incidence of cervical cancer is much more striking, with 83% of cervical cancers presenting in developing countries. Worldwide, 510,000 women will be diagnosed with cervical cancer each year. The highest incidence rates are observed in sub-Saharan Africa, Melanesia, Latin America, the Caribbean, and within south-central and southeast Asia. The large burden of disease is likely due to the lack of cancer prevention programs within developing countries.

Infection by high-risk HPV types can lead to both low- and high-grade changes within cervical cells. The evolution from infection by HPV, to development of a persistent infection, to precancerous transformation, to outright cervical cancer has been estimated to take 20 years or longer. This relatively slow progression is at the root of the success of cervical cancer screening programs.

32. How is cervical cancer staged?

Cervical cancer is staged based on clinical findings. The surgeon may recommend examination in the operating room under anesthesia (EUA) to get a better sense of your stage. The staging system is listed in **Table 2**.

HPV and Cervical Cancer

Table 2 Overview of Cervical Cancer Staging

Stage	Clinical Findings
0	Cancer in situ
I	Cancer is at the cervix only IA: Found by microscopic exam only IA1: ≤ 3.0 mm deep and ≤ 7.0 mm horizontally IA2: 3.0–5.0 mm deep and ≥ 7.0 mm horizontally IB: Clinically visible cancer IB1: Tumor is ≤ 4.0 cm IB2: Tumor is > 4.0 cm
II	Tumor extends beyond the uterus IIA: No parametrial invasion IIB: Parametrial invasion
III	Tumor extends to pelvic wall and/or involves the lower third of the vagina and/or causes blockage of the ureters IIIA: Tumor involves the lower third of the vagina without extension to the pelvic wall IIIB: Tumor extends to the pelvic wall and affects the kidneys or ureters, or else a tumor of any size involving the lymph nodes of the pelvis
IVA	Tumor invades the mucosa of the bladder or rectum, and/or extends beyond the true pelvis
IVB	Distant metastasis including to the nodes involving the para-aortic area

33. How is cervical cancer treated?

Cervical cancer treatment is dependent on your stage. Treatment may include removal of the cervix only, called a **trachelectomy**, if the disease is only microscopically visible and/or if the woman wants to try to have children in the future; radical hysterectomy, where the uterus and surrounding structures (called the parametrium) are removed; or lymph node dissection. If the cervical disease is over 2 inches in size—also referred to as bulky—then your doctor may recommend that treatment be medical with the use of chemotherapy and radiation. However, disease that has spread beyond

Trachelectomy

Treatment that involves removal of the cervix only.

the pelvis is not curable and chemotherapy may be used to control symptoms only.

34. Is cervical cancer curable?

Fortunately, the vast majority of women diagnosed with cervical cancer are cured because the disease can be caught early. Still, it is responsible for approximately 3500 deaths annually in the United States. Worldwide, it is a much larger problem, with 280,000 people dying of the disease each year. As cervical cancer becomes more advanced, the chances of cure go down. Disease limited to the pelvis is treated with chemotherapy and radiation with the aim to cure. However, once the disease leaves the pelvis, it is no longer a curable condition, and efforts to maintain quality of life and treat the cancer must be considered carefully.

Disease limited to the pelvis is treated with chemotherapy and radiation with the aim to cure.

PART SIX

HPV and Vaginal Cancer

What are the risks for vaginal cancer?

How is vaginal cancer diagnosed?

How is vaginal cancer treated?

More . . .

35. What is vaginal cancer?

Vaginal cancer is a rare cancer of the female pelvic tract that begins in the external area of the reproductive system. It involves cancer of the vaginal tissue.

36. How common is vaginal cancer?

There are two main types of vaginal cancers, with the glandular type adenocarcinomas more common in women under age 20 years and squamous cell cancers more common as a woman ages.

Primary cancers of the vagina are rare and account for just over 2000 cases each year, with only 800 deaths annually. Vaginal cancer accounts for 1–2% of all gynecologic cancers in the United States and less than 1% of all gynecologic cancers in the world. Given how rare it is, a diagnosis of primary cancer of the vagina is made by making sure that the cancer did not start somewhere else, such as the vulva or the cervix. This is especially true in women with a personal history of other cancers. There are two main types of vaginal cancers, with the glandular type *adenocarcinomas* more common in women under age 20 years and squamous cell cancers more common as a woman ages.

37. What are the risks for vaginal cancer?

The risk factors identified include both biological and social factors. The social factors include low educational level and low family income levels. Biologic factors include a prior history of abnormal Pap smears, genital warts, and vaginal discharge or irritation. A case-control study from Denmark also identified the risk factors for squamous cell carcinomas, of which detectable high-risk HPV DNA was one. Other risk factors included a prior history of cervical neoplasia, poor genital hygiene, tobacco smoking, and alcohol consumption. In one study, HPV was detected in 100% of specimens presenting with VAIN-1, 90% of those with VAIN-2, and 70% of those with vaginal carcinomas. A rare type of vaginal cancer is termed clear cell carcinoma. This type of vaginal cancer is very aggressive, and the predominant risk is if your mother was exposed to diethylstilbestrol (DES) while she was pregnant. In women with DES-associated vaginal cancer, the diagnosis tends to occur before the age of 20 years.

38. What is VAIN? Is it cancer?

No, VAIN is not cancer. It is a precancerous lesion known as vaginal intraepithelial neoplasia. Women are usually not symptomatic with it, and it is termed the same way cervical intraepithelial neoplasia (CIN) is described, using grades 1 through 3, depending on how the cells appear under the microscope. As in CIN, the higher the grade number, the more worrisome the lesion.

39. How is vaginal cancer diagnosed?

Vaginal cancer requires a biopsy of any identified suspicious areas. To help with this, colposcopy is usually required. The same solution used to detect abnormalities of the cervix, Lugol's solution, can also be applied to the vagina to assist your healthcare provider in biopsying the area of concern. Topical solution or silver nitrate is applied to the biopsy site to control bleeding.

40. How is vaginal cancer staged?

Vaginal cancers are staged by clinical examination. The system is noted in **Table 3**.

41. How is vaginal cancer treated?

Treatment is dictated by the extent of disease and the patient's age, although excision is generally regarded as the standard of care. Early disease is managed by surgical removal of the upper vagina, called a vaginectomy. This may be performed with hysterectomy if the

Table 3   Overview of Vaginal Cancer Staging

Stage	Description
0	Intraepithelial neoplasia (VAIN)
I	Cancer is limited to the vaginal wall
II	Carcinoma extends to subvaginal tissue but not to the pelvic wall
III	Carcinoma involves pelvic wall
IVA	Tumor invades bladder and/or rectal mucosa and/or directly extends beyond the true pelvis
IVB	Distant metastases

uterus is still present. The lymph nodes may also be removed by the surgeon at the same time.

Nonsurgical options include topical chemotherapy or laser surgery to remove the area of concern.

If surgery would be too risky because of your age or other illnesses, your doctor may recommend treatment without surgery, in which case chemotherapy and radiation may be used.

If there is no invasive cancer, and only VAIN, surgery may not be necessary as initial treatment. Nonsurgical options include topical chemotherapy or laser surgery to remove the area of concern.

PART SEVEN

HPV and Vulvar Cancer

What is vulvar cancer?

What are the risk factors for vulvar cancer?

What is the primary treatment for vulvar cancer?

More . . .

42. What is vulvar cancer?

The **vulva** comprises part of the external female genital system. It is the outermost area and connects the vagina to the outside of the body. The vulva includes the inner and outer lips of the vagina, the clitoris (the sensitive tissues between the lips), and the opening of the vagina and its glands. Cancers that begin here are termed vulvar cancer. The vast majority of vulvar cancers are squamous cell cancers.

Vulva

Part of the external female genital system. It connects the vagina to the outside of the body, and includes the inner and outer lips of the vagina, the clitoris (the sensitive tissues between the lips), and the opening of the vagina and its glands.

Vulvar cancer most often affects the outer vaginal lips. Less often, cancer affects the inner vaginal lips or the clitoris. Vulvar cancer usually develops slowly over a period of years because cells that are abnormal can grow on the surface of the vulvar skin for a long time. This precancerous condition is called **vulvar intraepithelia neoplasia (VIN)** or dysplasia. Because it is possible for VIN or dysplasia to develop into vulvar cancer, treatment of this condition is very important.

Vulvar cancer usually develops slowly over a period of years because cells that are abnormal can grow on the surface of the vulvar skin for a long time.

43. How do women present with vulvar cancer?

Vulvar intraepithelia neoplasia (VIN)

Precancerous condition also known as dysplasia.

Women often present with vulvar cancer after finding a lump in their genital area or once they start experiencing pain or itching. Some women do not have any symptoms. Vulvar cancer also can arise from a mole or some other lesion, so it is very important to carefully monitor any lesion or mole on the vulva. Often a biopsy is warranted. Unfortunately, given that these symptoms are quite common, diagnosis is often delayed. If you begin experiencing problems, however, it emphasizes the importance of the physical exam. Be certain to seek professional medical care to have your vulva examined carefully should you notice any lesions or warts.

44. How big a problem is vulvar cancer?

Cancer of the vulva is quite rare and comprises only 5% of the tumors coming from the female genital system. In the United States, 3700 women are diagnosed each year, and fewer than 900 deaths are reported.

Vulvar cancer also occurs at two peak ages in women. Young women can develop vulvar cancer; these lesions often are associated with HPV. In older women, vulvar cancer can develop independent of HPV. Estimates indicate that about 40% of cases worldwide are attributable to HPV infection.

45. What are the risk factors for vulvar cancer?

Beyond age, risk factors include the number of sexual partners you have had; history of genital warts; abnormal cervical cytology or other HPV-associated cancers; and smoking and a compromised immune system, whether due to drugs or infection such as HIV.

46. Is there a precancerous lesion of the vulva?

Yes, this precancerous lesion is called vulvar intraepithelial neoplasia (VIN). Vulvar intraepithelial neoplasia is classified into two broad categories: usual and differentiated. VIN, usual type, is associated with HPV infection. It is considered to be the precursor lesion to invasive vulvar carcinoma. However, VIN, differentiated type, is a more worrisome lesion that can be associated with frank vulvar cancer. It tends to occur in older women and presents as a single mass. It also has gradations of severity as well from worrisome to those having serious cellular changes.

Vulvar intraepithelial neoplasia is classified into two broad categories: usual and differentiated.

47. How is VIN treated?

Excision by surgery is the primary treatment for VIN, with the goal being to completely remove it without evidence at the surgical borders.

If the surgeon is sure there is no invasion (based on a diagnostic biopsy), then laser ablation using carbon dioxide is effective. However, treatment, particularly of multifocal lesions, can be associated with significant post-procedure pain, and healing may take a significant time.

For VIN, usual type, imiquimod has been used as a topical agent. In one study, more than 80% of those treated with imiquimod had a reduction in the size of their vulvar lesion and 58% of those on treatment cleared HPV from their lesion. After 12 months of follow-up, only one woman under treatment had progression to invasive carcinoma. The side effects from this medication can include local redness and irritation.

48. How is vulvar cancer staged?

Vulvar cancer is staged by clinical exam. The Fédération Internationale de Gynécologie et d'Obstétrique (FIGO) System is used (see **Table 4**).

49. What is the primary treatment for vulvar cancer?

Surgery is the primary treatment for vulvar cancer, but whether this method can be used depends on how extensive the disease is when found. A large surgery called a radical vulvectomy was once required to treat

Table 4 Overview of Vulvar Cancer Staging

Stage	Description
I	Lesion ≤ 2.0 cm confined to vulva or perineum No evidence of nodal involvement
IA	Lesion ≤ 2.0 cm confined to vulva and/or perineum; stromal invasion present but ≤ 1.0 mm No evidence of nodal involvement
II	Tumor confined to vulva and/or perineum >2.0 cm in greatest dimension No nodal metastases
III	Tumor of any size with: (i) lower urethra, vagina, and/or anal involvement; and/or (ii) unilateral regional nodes involved
IVA	Tumor invades any pelvic structures (upper urethra, bladder mucosa, rectal mucosa, pelvic bone) and/or bilateral node involvement
IVB	Distant metastases, including the pelvic nodes

vulvar cancer, in which the lymph nodes (which drain the vulva) also were removed. This surgery required a long recovery time with risks of complications after surgery and long-term risk of leg swelling, called lymphedema, due to the removal of all the lymph nodes. This surgery also was associated with sexual complaints, decreased sexual desire, and/or sexual pain syndromes.

Given the difficulties of surgery, conservative treatment of the area of concern is becoming more common. For smaller lesions, the control rate is excellent. The use of less aggressive pelvic node removal also has been championed, and recent studies have shown no detriment to survival with vast improvements in both short- and long-term complications.

HPV and Vulvar Cancer

If surgery is not an option, radiation with chemotherapy often is recommended. However, the use of primary chemotherapy with radiation is still under investigation, as currently, it is unclear whether the results are as good as surgical results. Still, our experience in treating cervical cancer makes it a reasonable option for a patient unable to proceed with surgery.

PART EIGHT

HPV and Penile Cancer

How is penile cancer diagnosed?

What are symptoms of penile cancer?

Can penile cancer be prevented?

More . . .

50. What is cancer of the penis?

A malignant growth that begins in a man's penis is called primary **penile cancer**. Penile cancers can begin anywhere on the penis, with about 50% involving the head of the penis (or glans) and 21% involving the foreskin (or prepuce). Penile cancer is rare in the developed world and accounts for 0.2% of cancers in U.S. males. However, in some countries of Africa and South America, it accounts for up to 10% of cancers in men.

Penile cancer is rare in the developed world and accounts for 0.2% of cancers in U.S. males.

51. What are the symptoms of penile cancer?

Penile cancer often presents early because the symptoms are alarming and are difficult to ignore. Redness, irritation, or a non-healing sore on the penis are some common symptoms, while others may present with a mass or lump on the penile tip or shaft. If you have any of these symptoms, it is important to seek medical care immediately.

52. How common is penile cancer?

Approximately 1300 men are diagnosed each year, and about 300 will die of penile cancer. Circumcised men rarely develop this type of cancer. It is estimated that approximately 40% of all cases of penile cancers are attributable to HPV infection.

53. How is penile cancer diagnosed?

Unfortunately, there is often a delay in medical attention for penile cancers, likely due to patient embarrassment, ignorance, or personal neglect. However, delays may also be due to physician ignorance of the disease. This often leads to trials of various ointments or topical creams to treat an atypical dermatitis.

Typically, men will present complaining of a sore that does not heal, subtle rash, or growth on the penis. At later stages, the cancer can look more like a nonhealing ulcer with bloody or infected borders.

Ultimately, the diagnosis is generally made by examination. If cancer is suspected, it will require a biopsy of the abnormal area.

54. How is it staged?

Unlike female cancers, penile cancers are staged using the American Joint Committee on Cancer (AJCC) staging system. This employs the use of criteria to define what the tumor looks like (T), whether lymph nodes are involved (N), and whether distant metastases are present (M). The classification and staging system is given below:

Stage 0: TisN0M0 or TaN0M0

Stage I: T1N0M0

Stage II: T1N1M0 or T2N0-1M0

Stage III: T1-2N2M0 or T3N0-2M0

Stage IV: T4N0-2M0 or T1-4N3M0 or T1-4N0-3M1

Tumor (T) Criteria:

Tx: Primary tumor not evaluated

T0: No primary tumor found

Tis: Cancer in situ

Ta: Noninvasive verrucous carcinoma

T1: Tumor involves the connective tissue under the skin

T2: Tumor invades the deeper layers of the penis (Corpus spongiosum or Corpus cavernosum)

T3: Tumor invades the urethra or the prostate

T3: Tumor involves other adjacent organs

Nodes (N) Criteria:

Nx: Regional nodes not assessed

N0: Negative node involvement

N1: Involves the superficial inguinal node

N2: Involves multiple or bilateral superficial inguinal nodes

N3: Involves the deep inguinal or pelvic nodes

Metastases (M) Criteria:

Mx: No distant metastases assessed

M0: No metastatic disease

M1: Distant metastatic disease

55. How is penile cancer usually treated?

Surgery is the most common mode of treatment. One of the more common procedures is a microsurgical procedure called **Mohs surgery**. This entails a microscope during surgery that guides the removal of the abnormal tumor layer by layer, enabling the surgeon to remove as little normal tissue as possible. Other forms of surgery may use lasers or cryotherapy (freezing). For tumors less than 2 cm^2, circumcision may be all that is required. Evaluation of the lymph nodes in the groin is required during surgery, but fortunately, a sentinel node procedure is done routinely. This can spare the patient from undergoing a full groin node dissection, with its

Mohs surgery

Microsurgical surgery procedure that guides the removal of the abnormal tumor layer by layer.

For tumors less than 2 cm^2, circumcision may be all that is required.

associated long-term consequences, including leg lymphedema.

If the lesion is too large, surgical excision may be necessary. In advanced cases where even excision is not possible, a man may need to have his penis amputated. In all cases, further treatment with either chemotherapy or radiation may be recommended to increase the chance of cure.

56. Can penile cancer be prevented?

Circumsion often is considered to be an effective method of HPV prevention, therefore reducing the risk of penile cancer. There has been some debate over whether circumcision is a form of prevention. One study reported the lifetime risk of a man in the United States developing invasive penile cancer to be 1 in 600 if he is uncircumcised, while other studies have reported a 3- to 22-fold increased risk in men with their foreskin preserved. However, cross-country data have questioned this association. One study showed that the risk of penile cancer in countries with a low rate of circumcision, such as Sweden and Japan, is about the same as in the United States.

PART NINE

HPV and Anal Cancer

What is anal cancer? How common is it?

What are some signs or symptoms of anal cancer?

How is anal cancer diagnosed?

More . . .

57. What is anal cancer? How common is it?

Anal cancer is cancer involving the lowest portion of the gastrointestinal tract, representing the end of the large intestine. It does not involve the skin that surrounds the anus (also called the perianal region).

More than 5000 people are diagnosed with anal cancer each year; it is the cause of death for about 700 people per year. While more women were diagnosed with it, and more women died of disease than men in 2009, it affects both sexes. Worldwide, approximately 90% of anal cancers are related to HPV infection, and about 73% of cases are due to HPV 16 infection.

In the United States, the incidence of anal cancer is greatly increased among men who have sex with men and among those who are HIV-positive.

In the United States, the incidence of anal cancer is greatly increased among men who have sex with men and among those who are HIV-positive. For men and for women in general, there are approximately 2 diagnosed cases per 100,000 people. This incidence is 35 diagnosed cases per 100,000 people for homosexual men, and 70 diagnosed cases per 100,000 people for HIV-positive men. In total, there are approximately 4000 cases diagnosed each year, with 500 deaths. When researchers have compared women with anal cancer to women who do not have anal cancer, several risk factors have been identified: More than one sexual partner, anal intercourse, history of genital warts, and tobacco smoking are all associated with increased risk.

58. What are some signs or symptoms of anal cancer?

The symptoms of anal cancer are not specific to this disease. Still, if they are present, it should prompt you to go see a doctor. Pain or pressure in or around the anus is a common complaint, as is bleeding. Others may complain of itching or discharge, a bump in the anal area, a change in bowel patterns (usually as constipation or difficulty moving your stools), or swollen lymph nodes in the groin or around the anus. If you have any of these symptoms, it is imperative that you seek professional medical care as soon as possible.

59. How is anal cancer diagnosed?

Like cervical cancer, there may be an opportunity to catch precancerous lesions involving the anus because anal cancer appears to arise from high-grade anal lesions called intraepithelial neoplasia (AIN). These can be visualized using an anoscope at the transition zone where the anus and the rectum meet.

The diagnosis of anal cancer otherwise generally is made by physical exam. As part of the exam, a **digital rectal exam** is required. This requires your healthcare provider to place a glove on his or her hand, and using lubrication, insert his or her finger through the rectum to feel around the anus, checking for bleeding, if pain can be reproduced, and evaluating if there are lumps in the area. In addition, your healthcare provider may place a scope, called an anoscope or proctoscope, into this area to look at the anus or through the rectum. If there is suspicion of an invasive lesion or cancer, an endoanal ultrasound, which uses a probe inserted into the anus, can be used to evaluate the tissue that makes up and supports the anus. However, the ultimate diagnosis requires a biopsy of any abnormal areas.

Digital rectal exams (DREs) are recommended on a yearly basis for all men 50 years of age and older and for women as a routine part of their pelvic exam. Finding cancer early, however, depends on the location of the lesion; cancers that begin higher up in the anal canal

Digital rectal exam
Physical exam that requires a healthcare provider to place a glove on his or her hand, and using lubrication, insert his or her finger through the rectum to feel around the anus, checking for bleeding, if pain can be reproduced, and evaluating if there are lumps in the area.

may escape a DRE and present at a much later stage. Anal cancer is staged using the American Joint Committee on Cancer (AJCC) Tumor, Node, and Metastases (TNM) system.

Stage 0: Carcinoma in situ (TisN0M0)

Stage I: T1N0M0

Stage II: T2 or T3; N0M0

Stage III:

IIIA: T1-3N1M0 or T4N0M0

IIIB: T4N1M0 or T(any)N2-3M0

Stage IV: T(any)N(any)M1

Tumor (T) Criteria:

Tx: Primary tumor cannot be assessed

T0: No primary tumor identified

Tis: Carcinoma in situ

T1: Tumor is up to 2 cm in span

T2: Tumor is 2–5 cm in span

T3: Tumor is greater than 5 cm in span

T4: Tumor invades local tissue (vagina, urethra, or bladder)

Nodes (N) Criteria:

Nx: Regional nodes not assessed

N0: No evidence of regional node involvement

N1: Spread to nodes around rectum

N2: Spread to nodes on one side of the groin or pelvis

N3: Spread to nodes near the rectum and pelvis or groin; or nodes on both groins or pelvic area are involved

Metastases (M) Criteria:

Mx: Distant involvement not assessed

M0: No distant spread

M1: Spread of cancer to other organs or nodes is identified

60. How is anal cancer treated?

This depends on how extensive the cancer is when it is found. Surgery to remove the cancer can be performed if it is local without evidence of spread. However, if it appears that the surgery will leave a **colostomy**—meaning the stool is diverted from its normal route of exit through the anus to instead exit through a stoma in the abdominal wall, to which a bag is placed—you may instead be a candidate for primary chemotherapy and radiation.

Colostomy

Procedure in which stool must be diverted from its normal route of exit through the anus to instead exit through a stoma in the abdominal wall, to which a bag is placed.

PART TEN

HPV and Head and Neck Cancers

What is the association of HPV and head and neck cancers?

What are the signs and symptoms of head and neck cancers?

How are head and neck cancers staged?

More . . .

61. What is a cancer of the head and neck?

Head and neck cancers are a group of diseases that begin in the head region. These include cancers of the oral cavity (including those that begin on the lips, gums, cheeks, the top of the mouth, and near the jawbone), sinuses and nasal cavity, the **pharynx** (the tube connecting the mouth to the esophagus), the voicebox (or larynx), and the lymph nodes in the head and neck. They account for 3–5% of cancers in the United States.

Pharynx

The tube connecting the mouth to the esophagus.

62. What is the association of HPV and head and neck cancers?

According to some articles, oral cancer and HPV is a new health concern. Although most mouth and throat cancers are associated with tobacco use and/or alcohol, studies have begun to show that HPV may be another major source of risk. HPV seems to be particularly strongly associated with cancer of the tonsils, although it is also found in biopsy samples at other nearby sites.

HPV seems to be particularly strongly associated with cancer of the tonsils.

How does a sexually transmitted virus become associated with cancers located so far away from the genitals? The answer is probably oral sex. Several studies have shown a relationship between oral sex and the presence of HPV DNA in mouth and throat samples. Other studies have shown a relationship between oral sex and HPV-positive throat cancers, particularly in those individuals who perform oral sex on men.

Taken as a group, these studies are yet another reminder that oral sex may not be considered completely safer sex. Some other sexually transmitted diseases can be spread by oral sex, including herpes, gonorrhea, Chlamydia, and syphilis. The use of condoms and practicing safer sex should therefore be used for oral sex as well as vaginal and anal sex. This is particularly true for individuals with infections such as HIV or herpes simplex, since both viruses have been shown to predispose people to acquiring HPV.

HPV, particularly HPV 16, seems to play a role in the development of a significant number of cancers of the mouth and throat. Oral sex increases the risk of acquiring an HPV infection in your mouth or throat. Although study results are mixed, it seems possible that smoking and alcohol use may interact with an HPV infection to increase the risk of cancer.

While this assoiciation has been identified, recent data from Johns Hopkins suggest that patients with HPV-positive head and neck cancers may survive longer than those whose tumors are not HPV-positive.

63. What are the signs and symptoms of head and neck cancers?

The symptoms depend on where the cancers are. Cancers beginning in the mouth can present with a lump or nonhealing sore, bleeding, or pain. Those involving the sinuses tend to present with a sinus infection that refuses to get better, even with antibiotics; trouble with the eyes; pain when eating; or bleeding. Cancers involving the pharynx can present with persistent ear pain.

64. How are head and neck cancers diagnosed?

A physical exam of the oral cavity is required to diagnose head and neck cancers, and if something abnormal is found, a biopsy is required. Your doctor may require additional tests to see how extensive the cancer is when found and to make sure they know the extent of the cancer at diagnosis.

65. How are head and neck cancers staged?

The AJCC TNM system is used to stage cancers of the head and neck.

Stage 0: TisN0M0

Stage I: T1N0M0

Stage II: T2N0M0

Stage III: T3N0M0 or T1-3N1M0

Stage IV:

IVA: T4aN0-1M0; T1-2N2M0, T3-T4aN2M0

IVB: T4bN(any)M0, T(any)N3M0

IVC: T(any)N(any)M1

Primary Tumor (T)

Tx: Primary tumor cannot be assessed

T0: No evidence of primary tumor

Tis: Carcinoma in situ

Supraglottis (Above the Vocal Cords)

T1: Tumor limited to one area of the supraglottis; vocal cords are normal

T2: Tumor invades mucosa of supraglottis, glottis, or region outside the supraglottis (e.g., mucosa of base of tongue, vallecula, or medial wall of pyriform sinus) without involvement of the larynx

T3: Tumor limited to the larynx with vocal cord paralysis and/or invades other local areas

T4: Locally advanced

> T4a: Tumor invades the thyroid cartilage and/or invades beyond the larynx (e.g., trachea, soft tissues of the neck including deep extrinsic muscle of the tongue, strap muscles, thyroid, or esophagus)

> T4b: Tumor invades prevertebral space, encases the carotid artery, or invades the mediastinum

Glottis

T1: Tumor limited to the vocal cord(s)

> T1a: Tumor limited to one vocal cord

> T1b: Tumor involves both vocal cords

T2: Tumor extends to supraglottis and/or subglottis, and/or involves impaired vocal cord mobility

T3: Tumor limited to the larynx with vocal cord fixation and/or invades paraglottic space, and/or involves minor thyroid cartillage

T4: Locally advanced

> T4a: Tumor invades the thyroid cartilage and/or invades tissues beyond the larynx

> T4b: Tumor invades prevertebral space, encases carotid artery, or invades mediastinal structures

Subglottis

T1: Tumor limited to the subglottis

T2: Tumor extends to vocal cord(s) with normal or impaired mobility

T3: Tumor limited to larynx with vocal cord fixation

T4: Locally advanced

T4a: Tumor invades cricoid or thyroid cartilage and/or invades tissues beyond the larynx

T4b: Tumor invades prevertebral space, encases carotid artery, or invades mediastinum

Regional Lymph Nodes (N)

Nx: Regional lymph nodes cannot be assessed

N0: No regional lymph node metastasis

N1: Metastasis in a single ipsilateral lymph node up to 3 cm in greatest dimension

N2: Metastasis in a single ipsilateral lymph node 3–6 cm or smaller in greatest dimension, or in multiple ipsilateral lymph nodes with largest no more than 6 cm, or in bilateral or contralateral lymph nodes with all nodes less than 6 cm in greatest dimension

N2a: Metastasis in a single ipsilateral lymph node between 3 and 6 cm in greatest dimension

N2b: Metastasis in multiple ipsilateral lymph nodes 6 cm or smaller in greatest dimension

N2c: Metastasis in bilateral or contralateral lymph nodes 6 cm or smaller in greatest dimension

N3: Metastasis in a lymph node larger than 6 cm in greatest dimension

Distant Metastasis (M)

MX: Distant metastasis cannot be assessed

M0: No distant metastasis

M1: Distant metastasis

66. How are head and neck cancers treated?

Treatment will largely depend on the extent of disease when it is found. If found early enough, surgery may be considered curative. However, in an effort to spare organ function (i.e., ability to eat and talk), primary treatment may consist of chemotherapy and radiation. Treatment can be quite toxic, and you may need a feeding tube during treatment due to the swelling and tissue breakdown that is expected with treatment.

HPV and Head and Neck Cancers

PART ELEVEN

Prevention and Education

Can condoms prevent HPV spread?

What should I tell my partner about being HPV positive?

For women, how often should Pap smears be performed?

More . . .

67. Can condoms prevent HPV spread?

Recent published data on condom use suggests that there may be limited to no protection against HPV infection and transmission. There is some indication that the disease may be less likely to cause symptoms amongst condom users. Because HPV is not transmitted in semen or body fluids but rather through direct skin-to-skin contact, HPV infections are not theoretically prevented with condoms since the extent of skin that could be infected extends beyond the area that is typically covered by a condom. This is not to say that condoms do not protect against other very dangerous sexually transmitted diseases (STDs); latex condoms are very effective for protection against HIV infection. Men and women who are sexually active in ways other than long-term monogamous relationships must use condoms to help reduce sexually transmitted diseases such as gonnorhea, clamydia, hepatitis, and HIV. Despite the theoretical reason against condom protection for HPV, it is worth noting that the CDC recommends using condoms as a way to reduce the risk of HPV infection.

The CDC recommends using condoms as a way to reduce the risk of HPV infection.

If you are involved in a long-term relationship with someone who is HPV infected, it is very likely that you are already infected too. In this case, it is very important that health screening include examination of the anal and genital areas. You should be vigilant and check yourself for the appearance of warts or other concerning changes. Seek professional medical care from a specialist to ensure that genital areas are inspected and that warts are identified and treated early and effectively.

Carol says:

Some patients are completely flabbergasted when they find out they have an HPV infection because they've always practiced safe sex with condoms. General questions about condom use and effectiveness quickly surface. The fact that only 30% of HPV infections may be prevented with condom use doesn't offer much support.

The common perspective of STD transmitted diseases is based on the idea that they're transmitted by body fluids for which condoms are used. But in the case of HPV, the explanation that skin regions outside the condom-protected area may harbor the virus, quickly makes sense of the picture. It's possible that intercourse may not occur and yet HPV has been transmitted from one person to another by skin contact in genital friction.

That's not a reason to discontinue using condoms, though. Condoms are very useful in preventing pregnancy and contracting other STD's. And, when it comes to preventing HPV transmission by condoms, reducing the risk of infection by 30% is still worth it. Thinking that you have a 30% chance (nearly one in three) of winning something is convincing to try it.

68. What should I tell my partner about being HPV positive?

Whether to talk to your sexual partner about HPV positivity and, for women, their Pap test results, is a personal decision. Remember that most adults will get one or more types of HPV if they are or have been in a sexual relationship. Chances are, your partner had already been exposed to HPV by the time your infection was detected. If you are in a monogamous relationship, there is no risk of passing the infection back and forth. Once you "share" a particular strain of the virus through sexual contact, you cannot be re-infected with the same type. When you are sexually active with a new partner, use of a condom—although it doesn't provide complete protection—can help prevent the spread of HPV and other STDs.

Another important concern is that it is impossible to know for certain from whom you originally received the HPV virus. You may have been exposed in a relationship months or years earlier, and the infection may have been dormant, or "silent," in the meantime. Trying to determine who is at fault is not possible or productive, and it may cause unnecessary stress. You may not have gotten it from your current partner; blaming him or her is unproductive. Self-guilt or shame is not helpful either.

The best policy is to be open and honest with your partner. Remember, everyone who is or has been sexually active is at risk for, or has been infected with, HPV.

Carol says:

After the initial questions about what HPV infection means, a range of emotions is common—from fear and embarrassment, to disgust and anger. The discussion can be charged with hints of blame or obvious anger towards the partner.

At this point, these emotions need to be re-directed because the variables of an HPV infection, the "who, when, and where" of the situation, can be unclear and useless. The primary focus is returning to good health.

What you tell your partner is a personal decision. Remember that the chances are pretty good if you have it, so does your partner. One factor most often considered is how the partner is emotionally built, since the discussion can result in the initial reaction that you had. Understanding how HPV operates can also affect the decision. Thinking about how you would like to be treated if the roles were reversed can also help in the decision about what to share. Regardless of the choice, the plan to return to good health through protection and prevention will benefit you and your partner.

69. I would like to prevent HPV-associated cancers—what can I do?

Different organizations and various task forces periodically publish patient care guidelines about how people should be screened for a specific disease. For example, the American Cancer Society, American College of Obstetricians and Gynecologists, and other associations, such as the U.S. Preventative Services Task Force, American College of Cardiology, and American Association of Gastrointestinal Surgeons, all produce various age-specific guidelines as to how often women should be screened. Many of these guidelines are conflicting and may be confusing, so it is best to formulate a healthcare plan with your trusted healthcare team. Different women are at risk for differing cancers, so it is best to individualize your plan.

The bottom line is that care needs to be tailored to a woman's specific history and medical needs. For women who have had pelvic surgery for cancer, Pap test screening of the vaginal cuff is recommended, even if the cervix, uterus, and ovaries have been removed. Typically, the primary care provider (gynecologist or internist) or gynecologic oncologist will perform these for several years after cancer treatment to ensure that the cancer is not recurring.

Because there is no recommended screening test to detect vulvar or vaginal cancer, it is important to note if a woman has any unusual symptoms, including itchiness, burning in the vulvar area, dry scaly skin, bleeding, or abnormal discharge from the vulvar area, she should report these changes to her healthcare provider and may need an outpatient biopsy to get a definitive diagnosis of the troubling area. The rule of thumb is to have a biopsy if there is anything abnormal on the vulva.

The rule of thumb is to have a biopsy if there is anything abnormal on the vulva.

The vulva is known as the great mimicker. Many lesions can look similar, and the general rule is to biopsy a suspicious lesion. Women also can perform self vulvar examinations with the aid of a hand-held mirror and report any changes in skin color or surface texture to their doctor. Any lesion that has changes in area, border, color, or diameter (ABCD) should be reported to the healthcare provider and biopsied. Many cancer institutions have functionalized screening programs so regular visits can be scheduled every 6 months with a healthcare provider.

Presently there are no medically recommended or approved screening tests for HPV for men, and none are routinely preformed. Maintaining a strong sense of personal vigilance for signs of a problem are important; self-exam may be helpful. Signs of infection may include a nonhealing rash, ulcerations on the skin (particularly on the penis, testicles, or anus), pain when urinating or defecating, bleeding, or swollen genitopelvic glands.

For all patients, prevention also should concentrate on removal of other factors that may work with HPV to increase risk. In particular, the importance of avoidance and/or stopping smoking is essential, as it is a significant cofactor in the development of disease caused by HPV. Safer sex practices are always encouraged, and the liberal use of condoms to prevent other serious diseases is always recommended.

Carol says:

With the estimated number of sexually active people exposed to HPV being 75%, prevention falls into two categories: before and after the first exposure.

In the "before" exposure group, HPV vaccination for up to 70% protection is considered if the girl is between age 11–26.

The "after" exposure group shares five other prevention strategies with the "before group". These include:

1. *Practicing safe sex may prevent 30% of HPV infections.*
2. *Limiting the number of sex partners–the fewer the better.*
3. *Stopping smoking—HPV and smoking are positively linked to cervical cancer. Quitting smoking breaks this link.*
4. *Building a healthy immune system by eating a balanced diet, getting adequate sleep, and including exercise.*
5. *Scheduling regular gynecologic appointments for screening.*

The positive message is that although there is no single method to guarantee HPV prevention, there are several steps you can take to limit the chances that HPV will affect your health!

70. For women, how often should Pap smears be performed?

The American College of Obstetricians and Gynecologists recently revised their recommendations for Pap tests. They now recommend that Pap tests be done once a woman reaches the age of 21, regardless of whether or not, or how long, she has been sexually active. Screening should then be performed every 2 years until age 30. If a woman in her 30s is in a stable monogamous relationship and has had negative Pap tests and no risk factors for getting HPV, then screening can happen every 3 years. Recent advances in science have combined testing of the Pap test with another test for high-risk HPV. If both are negative, then repeat testing using this combination every 3 years also is reasonable. For women who have had a hysterectomy due to noncancerous reasons, Pap tests may be discontinued. However, if personal history changes and you are at an increased risk for developing cervical changes, you should switch back to being screened annually. Aspects of your social behavior may influence the interval of Pap screening, such as if you get divorced and are now dating multiple people, or if a partner is diagnosed with dysplasia or warts.

These guidelines do not pertain to women with other special medical conditions who may be at a higher risk for cervical changes or cancer. These include women with HIV, women on medicines that affect the immune system, or those who have a prior history of cervical cancer.

71. Do these guidelines extend to older women?

Women over 70 years of age who have had three negative Pap tests in a row and no history of abnormal Pap tests in the prior 10 years may not need continued screening and can discuss stopping screening with their healthcare providers. Just because you have discontinued having Pap smears does not mean you do not need to see your gynecologist—you still need to have an annual pelvic examination of the vulva, vagina, and other pelvic structures that can develop pathology. Discontinuing cervical screening occurs because cervical cancer is rare among older women who have been screened, and the quality of the samples that are taken as a woman ages decreases due to the physical changes in the vagina and the cervix.

72. Are people who are HIV infected followed differently?

In people living with HIV, HPV plays a large role in the development of cancers involving the cervix and anus. Women infected with HIV should undergo a Pap test twice the first year after they are diagnosed, and then annually, provided that the prior tests were normal. Some doctors will recommend a frequency of testing dependent on a woman's T-cell count.

If a woman does have abnormal cells, she should be followed carefully. Other women who are immuno-compromised or are at increased risk for cervical cancer because their mother took a drug called diesthylstilbe-strol (DES) while pregnant should be screened annually as well, even if prior Pap tests are normal. These women are at increased risk for developing other cancers such as clear cell carcinoma.

Men with HIV are at an increased risk of anal cancers, and for these patients, some medical professionals advocate Pap smears of the anal canal (mentioned in more detail in Question 15). While it has yet to be established that screening reduces the risk or incidence of anal cancers, some centers have started screening HIV-positive men at 6–12 month intervals with recommendations for more invasive procedures (anoscopy and biopsy) if AIN is found. More data, including formalized guidelines, have yet to be established.

73. If I have had my uterus removed, do I still need to have Pap tests?

If you have had your uterus removed (called a **hysterectomy**) for noncancer-related reasons, such as **fibroids**

HPV plays a large role in the development of cancers involving the cervix and anus.

Hysterectomy
Removal of the uterus.

Fibroids
Noncancerous muscle outgrowths from the uterus.

(noncancerous muscle outgrowths from the uterus), excessive bleeding, or endometriosis, there is no reason to have Pap tests performed. However, if you had a hysterectomy due to cancer of the cervix, vagina, vulva, ovaries, or uterus, you should continue to be screened. As discussed previously, you still need to see your healthcare provider on an annual basis for a complete examination and monitoring of the pelvic structures.

74. If I am pregnant, will being HPV-positive be a factor in the delivery of my baby?

Neonatal laryngeal papillomatosis

A type of HPV infection that can occur in the newborn baby with symptoms of warts in the throat or voice box.

While transmission from a mother to newborn has been reported, there is a very low risk for HPV transmission to the unborn baby during a vaginal delivery.

It was once recommended that women with genital warts (a type of HPV) be offered cesearean section (C-section) delivery if they went into labor to prevent **neonatal laryngeal papillomatosis**, a type of HPV infection that can occur in the newborn baby with symptoms of warts in the throat or voice box. If the warts are in the vagina, they can also make the vagina less elastic or even block the birth canal; if are large and block the birth canal, a C-section delivery may be necessary. However, HPV infection and genital warts are not the only reasons for having a C-section, as warts may grow and become large during pregnancy's possibly immunosuppressive time. HPV research scientists are not certain why in some cases genital warts grow during pregnancy. Female hormones, like estrogen and progesterone, a change in the environment, or changes in the immune system may play a role.

While transmission from a mother to newborn has been reported, there is a very low risk for HPV transmission to the unborn baby during a vaginal delivery. Fortunately, even when the virus is passed, most newborns are able to get rid of the virus on their own. In rare cases, a baby that is exposed to HPV may develop laryngeal papillomatosis. Although uncommon, this is a potentially life-threatening condition for the child, requiring frequent laser surgery to prevent obstruction of the breathing passages. These warts can occur up to 5 years after birth.

Carol says:

When pregnant women find out they're positive for HPV, two concerns surface: what it means for their delivery, and what the disease and its treatment may mean for the unborn baby while they're pregnant. It's reassuring for them that special considerations are made at these times.

While many of the standard medical treatments for warts are safe to use in pregnancy, podophyllin and interferon are not. Also, timing the treatment during the middle of the second half of pregnancy may be more successful. To be safe, a more cautious approach is used to treat cervical dysplasia. During pregnancy this type of infection is followed closely with pap smears or biopsies.

Delivery by C-section is based on several factors and is not an automatic decision just because a woman is HPV positive. In fact, babies born by C-section have also been found to have HPV. Regardless of the method of delivery, it's very rare that a baby is born with a serious HPV infection called laryngeal papillomatosis.

75. What is an anal Pap smear?

Anal Pap smears use the same techniques that are used in cervical Pap smears, but the test is applied to the anal mucosa. It is not a recommended screening test in men, nor is it recommended in women. However, some experts suggest such screening in gay, bisexual, HIV-positive, or otherwise immunocompromised people. During an anal Pap smear, a sampling of cells is taken using a Dacron swab of the surfaces of the anus and rectum. The cells are then analyzed by a microscope to see if any structural changes are present that may be precursors to cancer. Screening has been suggested every 3 years for gay and bisexual men, but again, this reflects some expert opinions and are not consensus recommendations. For HIV-positive men and women, the screening interval may be more frequently recommended.

PART TWELVE

HPV Vaccination: What You Should Know

What is the cervical cancer vaccine?

What are the side effects to the vaccine?

How do I cope with HPV?

More . . .

76. How do vaccines work?

Vaccines work by teaching the immune system to recognize and attack bacteria or viruses that can cause disease in the human body.

Vaccines work by teaching the immune system to recognize and attack bacteria or viruses that can cause disease in the human body. Many types of vaccines are administered today, most of which are administered beginning shortly after birth and continuing through young adulthood.

A **vaccine** is a method of training the body to recognize disease-causing bacteria or viruses by exposing the immune system to either a portion of the bacteria or virus, or to the whole bacteria or virus that has been made inactive, and thus unable to cause disease. A classic example of a vaccine that is made from an inactive virus is the polio vaccine. An example of a vaccine that is made from a replica of a portion of a virus is the hepatitis B vaccine. The hepatitis B vaccine is made by implanting the part of the hepatitis B virus DNA that causes growth of the hepatitis B virus shell into an animal cell. The animal cell then produces many copies of the shell of the virus without the active particle inside. Once it is injected, this shell is recognized by the immune system without the risk of contracting the actual disease and as such, the vaccine causes an immune response. Immune cells in the body learn to recognize the vaccine so that when a person is exposed to the real disease-causing bacteria or virus, the memory of how to respond is already prepared and the disease can be avoided.

Vaccination has had a huge impact on disease in the United States. For example, prior to vaccination for measles, there was almost 900,000 cases per year. Following the introduction of vaccination, it has been reduced to just 86 cases per year. Similar findings have

Vaccine

A method of training the body to recognize disease-causing bacteria or viruses by exposing the immune system to either a portion of the bacteria or virus, or to the whole bacteria or virus that has been made inactive.

occurred with widespread vaccination against mumps and whooping cough (also known as pertussis). On a global scale, it is estimated that vaccines help to prevent three million deaths each year.

77. What is the cervical cancer vaccine?

The cervical cancer vaccine has been developed to protect against certain types of human papilloma virus (HPV). There are two types of vaccines for use in the United States. One type protects against four different strains of HPV (quadrivalent), and the other protects against two strains of HPV (bivalent). The quadrivalent vaccine is called **Gardasil**, and was the first approved in the United States. The bivalent vaccine is **Cervarix**, which was approved in the US in 2009. A comparison of the two vaccines is given in Questions 78 and 79. Typically, three injections are needed; the intervals are discussed in **Table 5**.

On a global scale, it is estimated that vaccines help to prevent three million deaths each year.

Gardasil

Quadrivalent vaccine that protects against HPV types 6, 11, 16, and 18; the first approved in the United States.

Cervarix

Bivalent vaccine designed to protect against HPV 16 and 18; approved in some countries for use, but not in the United States.

Table 5   Cervical Cancer Vaccines

Characteristic	Quadrivalent	Bivalent
Trade name	Gardasil	Cervarix
Manufacturer	Merck	Glaxo Smith Kline
HPV types covered	6, 11, 16, 18	16, 18
Expression via	Yeast	Baculovirus
Schedule	0, 2, 6 months	0, 1, 6 months
U.S. FDA approved	Yes	Yes
Most common toxicity	Mild–moderate injection site symptoms (pain, swelling, redness, pruritis)	Injection site pain

78. What is Gardasil?

Gardasil is an inactive vaccine and there is no risk of becoming infected with HPV by receiving it. It is currently approved for use in girls as young as 9 years old and in women up to the age of 26. In 2009, the FDA also approved its use in males between the ages of 9 and 26. Between 2007 and 2008 it was estimated that up to 35% of adolescent girls had been vaccinated with at least one injection. It is important to know that even with vaccination, females still need to get Pap smears even if you have had the vaccine.

79. What is Cervarix?

Unlike Gardasil, Cervarix is a bivalent vaccine against HPV 16 and 18. It uses an aluminum salt formulation to boost the immune response. It is also approved for use in the United States, but its approval is limited for use in girls and women under the age of 26.

80. Will the vaccine mean women will not need to get Pap tests anymore?

The HPV vaccine is designed to prevent infection by HPV types 6, 11, 16, and 18. Unfortunately, there are many other HPV types that can infect the cervix, vagina, and vulva. These other HPV types can cause cervical cancer, genital warts, and other precancerous changes on the cervix, vagina, or vulva. For that reason, Pap tests are still recommended as a method of screening for these diseases. You also need to see a healthcare provider to make sure that your genitopelvic anatomy is healthy.

81. If I have been infected with HPV, will the vaccine protect me from getting cervical cancer?

The vaccine is only designed to be effective against HPV types 6, 11, 16, and 18. Some women infected with HPV may have one or more of these types. For example, if a woman has been infected with HPV type 18, the vaccine will not protect her against the effects of type 18. However, it will provide her protection against the other three types. The initial studies with these vaccines included some patients who had an infection with one or more of these HPV types. There was a definite benefit proven for these patients. Based on the evidence, the vaccine is recommended in women with a prior or current HPV infection.

Based on the evidence, the vaccine is recommended in women with a prior or current HPV infection.

82. How old do you have to be to be vaccinated? Can I be vaccinated if I am pregnant?

The current recommendations from the Advisory Committee on Immunization Practices recommends routinely vaccinating girls at 11–12 years of age. Vaccination can start as early as age 9 years, provided it is at the discretion of a healthcare provider. For older girls and women under age 27 years, vaccination also is recommended as "catch up," meaning that it is offered to older girls who may have delayed being vaccinated or were unable to be vaccinated at the recommended age.

Vaccination in pregnant women is not recommended. Although studies in rats of the currently available quadrivalent vaccine showed no harm to the fetus, and

phase III trials did not show any unintended consequences in women vaccinated versus those who had
received a placebo, the data on its use in pregnancy has
not been studied sufficiently. Therefore, current recommendations call for a delay in conception for at
least 30 days after the three-dose schedule has been
completed. If the series of shots has not been started,
then delay of vaccination is recommended until after
the pregnancy is completed. In a woman who discovers
she is pregnant but has already started the vaccine
series, completion of the shots should be delayed until
after delivery.

It is important to know that women who have had an
abnormal Pap smear or who are already sexually active
can be vaccinated. However, the protection against
HPV may be less than what is expected in a young girl
being vaccinated before she is sexually active.

83. What are the side effects of the vaccine?

The most common side effects of the current cervical
cancer vaccine are redness, swelling, and pain at the
injection site, similar to most vaccinations, headache,
fever, nausea, or vomiting. Fainting can occur after
vaccination, particularly among adolescents and young
adults. A small fraction of women may experience a
fever and flu-like symptoms. There have been a few
reports of patients being allergic to the vaccine. Some
patients may experience some light-headedness. In the
long-term follow-up of patients involved in the original trials, there have been no long-term side effects.

Allergic reactions that may occur include difficulty
breathing, wheezing (bronchospasm), hives, and rash.
Some of these reactions have been severe. Additional

side effects reported include swollen glands (neck, armpit, or groin), joint pain, or aching.

The HPV vaccine is contraindicated in pregnancy but not in lactating women. If a woman receives the vaccine and then discovers she is pregnant, she should report it to her healthcare provider as soon as possible. The healthcare provider should report it to the manufacturer. A registry of pregnant patients who have received the vaccine is being compiled to assess any effects on the developing fetus. To date, there have been no associated birth defects.

The HPV vaccine is contraindicated in pregnancy but not in lactating women.

84. Should men and boys get vaccinated? What if you are HIV-positive?

Yes. In 2009 the FDA approved Gardasil for vaccination in boys and men under the age of 26. The data is derived from studies in men. In one study of Gardasil on young men found that vaccination reduced the incidence of genital warts due to HPV 6, 11, 16, or 18 by 90%. There were also no incident diagnoses of penile or anal cancer in the vaccinated group, though this may not manifest for years. Currently, however, it is not recommended.

Given the high risk of HPV-associated cancers in HIV-positive men and women, this may be another potential use of the HPV vaccine. However, neither the safety or effectiveness in women with HIV is clear, and studies are currently underway. One of the issues has to do with the HPV types that cause cervical cancer in women with HIV. Some studies suggest that a greater range of HPV types are responsible for the disease; thus, HPV vaccination with the currently available vaccines would not be very effective.

85. Is the HPV vaccine linked to neurologic disease?

According to research presented at the American Academy of Neurology annual conference in Seattle, females who receive the vaccine do not have an increased risk of developing **Guillain Barre Syndrome**, a disorder where the immune system attacks the peripheral nerves, leading to paralysis.

Guillain Barre Syndrome

A disorder where the immune system attacks the peripheral nerves, leading to paralysis.

The data were analyzed from the 2006–2008 data bank on adverse events, and researchers found 36 cases of Guillain Barre Sydrome in girls and women aged 13–50 years after vaccination with Gardasil. Symptoms occurred within 6 weeks after vaccination in 75% of the cases. The researchers determined an incidence of Guillain Barre syndrome of about 7 per 1 million in the post-Gardasil population compared to 4.0–10.0 per 1 million in the general population. The researchers concluded that the syndrome did not occur more frequently in the HPV vaccination group.

86. How long are you protected after receiving the HPV vaccine?

The HPV vaccine is designed to offer lifetime protection from HPV. The question of whether a booster injection will be required remains to be answered. With more than 5 years of follow-up with the patients originally vaccinated in the trial, there has not yet been a need demonstrated for a booster vaccine.

The HPV vaccine is designed to offer lifetime protection from HPV.

The HPV vaccine is a three-injection series administered over a 6-month span. Although it is possible that some women will gain immunity after only one or two injections, it is unsafe to assume that a woman is protected until after she has completed the three-shot series.

87. Why should I get a vaccine if Pap tests are so effective?

Pap tests are a form of secondary cancer prevention. They do not address the fundamental causes of cervical cancer, the most common of which is HPV. The purpose of the HPV vaccine is **primary prevention**, or to prevent the *cause* of cervical cancer from infecting a patient.

Primary prevention
To prevent the cause of cervical cancer from infecting a patient; this is the purpose of the HPV vaccine.

Unfortunately, Pap tests are not a perfect test. Approximately 20% of women with cervical cancer will have had a recent false negative Pap test. This is by no means the fault of the healthcare provider obtaining the sample or the one interpreting the results. There is just an inherent lack of accuracy within the test that is only overcome because the test is repeated on a relatively frequent (annual) basis.

Another major problem with relying on Pap tests is compliance. This means not having the Pap test done at the recommended interval. This occurs either because the patient did not pursue it or there is a shortage of providers or funding to do the test for patients. Although never meant to replace the need for Pap tests, vaccination may help to address the worldwide problem of starting and continuing screening programs. In this way, it is hoped that vaccines can prevent a certain number of cancers annually, even for those unable or not willing to be screened.

Once you have been treated for HPV, the most important thing you can do for your health is to continue to have regular check-ups.

88. How do I cope with HPV?

Once you have been treated for HPV, the most important thing you can do for your health is to continue to have regular check-ups. If you have been recently diagnosed and treated, you will need more frequent exams to be sure that warts have been removed. After successful treatment, men and women should continue to examine their genitals regularly to check for warts and have annual physical exams to check for any new warts or growths that may not be visible. Women should also receive annual Pap smear tests to identify any cervical cell changes. Maintaining a healthy lifestyle is also important: limited alcohol, no tobacco, and a balanced diet. Getting a good night of rest, limiting stress, and a diet rich in antioxidants is also important. Include fruits, vegetables, and berries in your diet. Maintaining a healthy lifestyle will decrease the chances of HPV recurrences, and in time, most people stop having any recurrences.

You can reduce your risk of transmitting HPV to a sexual partner by abstaining from sex, by finding other ways to express intimacy, by avoiding contact with any wart, and/or by using condoms correctly and consistently every time you have sex. Like all safer sex methods (with the exception of abstinence), using condoms is not 100% safe—genital warts not covered by a condom can still transmit the virus, but condoms are still a crucial step to minimize risk for people who continue to be sexually active.

89. Can I ever have sex again?

Being diagnosed with HPV does not mean that you can never have sex again! It is important to communicate with your sexual partner(s) and give them information about HPV so they may make informed decisions about sexual activity.

Telling a partner that you have HPV, or any other type of sexually transmitted disease, can be a difficult, distressing, and challenging experience. Some partners may react by needing some time to think about how this affects your relationship. Others may have a lot of questions, and perhaps may get tested themselves.

It is completely normal to feel frustrated, depressed, angry, or guilty about having HPV. Sometimes sexual healthcare experts or counselors can help you cope with having a sexually transmitted disease. Many people who have HPV or other sexually transmitted infections may have the same concerns, and there also are support groups available.

By taking care of your health, practicing safer sex, and informing yourself and your partners, you are taking all the necessary steps to minimize the risk of recurrences and/or transmitting the virus to others.

Glossary

A

Adenocarcinoma: The second most common type of squamous cell carcinoma; indicates that the cancer arose within the glands of the cervix.

Anal cancer: Cancer involving the lowest portion of the gastrointestinal tract, representing the end of the large intestine.

Auto inoculation: Method of virus transmission that occurs when a person infects him- or herself.

C

Capsid: A shell that surrounds the virus, generally made up of proteins.

Cerclage: A stitch placed in the cervix after a woman has become pregnant to help strengthen the cervix for the remainder of the pregnancy.

Cervarix: Bivalent vaccine designed to protect against HPV 16 and 18; approved in some countries for use, but not in the United States.

Cervical cancer: Occurs when abnormal cells begin in the cervix and grow beyond their normal origin to become invasive.

Cervical dysplasia: Describes changes in the cells of the cervix, seen only under a microscope, that are precancerous lesions.

Cervical intraepithelial neoplasia (CIN): Another term for cervical dysplasia and is used to describe the findings on a cervical biopsy.

Colostomy: Procedure in which stool must be diverted from its normal route of exit through the anus to instead exit through a stoma in the abdominal wall, to which a bag is placed.

Colposcopy: A method of more closely evaluating a woman with an abnormal Pap test by using a high-powered microscope to view the cervix.

Cone biopsy: The most common surgery in women with suspicious findings from a colposcopy.

Cryotherapy: Surgical freezing of warts, usually using liquid nitrogen.

D

Digital rectal exam: Physical exam that requires a healthcare provider to place a glove on his or her hand, and using lubrication, insert his or her finger through the rectum to feel around the anus, checking for bleeding, if pain can be reproduced, and evaluating if there are lumps in the area.

Dormant: Inactive. Dormant viruses do not kill host cells.

E

Envelope: A membrane that surrounds a virus so it can live.

External genital warts (EGW): Commonly present as raised, peaked cauliflower-like lesions on the male or female genitalia. However, they can also be flat, rough or smooth.

F

Fibroids: Noncancerous muscle outgrowths from the uterus.

Flat warts: Warts on the face.

G

Gardasil: Quadrivalent vaccine that protects against HPV types 6, 11, 16, and 18; the only vaccine approved in the United States.

Genome: The complete genetic information of a virus or other organism.

Guillain Barre Syndrome: A disorder where the immune system attacks the peripheral nerves, leading to paralysis.

H

Human papilloma virus (HPV): A member of the family Papillomaviridae, Group I. It is a double-stranded DNA virus.

Hysterectomy: Removal of the uterus.

M

messenger RNA (mRNA): The blueprint by which proteins are produced.

Mohs surgery: Microsurgical surgery procedure that guides the removal of the abnormal tumor layer by layer.

N

Neonatal laryngeal papillomatosis: A type of HPV infection that can occur in the newborn baby with symptoms of warts in the throat or voice box.

P

Pap test (Pap smear): Test for women that enables a healthcare provider to test for changes in the cervix, which may be related to an infection with HPV.

Penile cancer: A malignant growth that begins in a man's penis.

Pharynx: The tube connecting the mouth to the esophagus.

Plantar warts: Warts on the soles of the foot.

Podophyllin: An antimitotic agent that works by stopping cells from growing.

Primary prevention: To prevent the cause of cervical cancer from infecting a patient; this is the purpose of the HPV vaccine.

R

Reflex HPV testing: Screens for the presence or absence of high-risk HPV typology when a cell test from a Pap smear is abnormal.

S

Squamous cells: The cells that make up the majority of the skin lining throughout the body, including the cervix.

T

T-cells: Immune cells that fight against viruses.

Taxonomy: Classification system based on the characteristics viruses have in common.

Trachelectomy: Treatment that involves removal of the cervix only.

Transformation zone: The place where the glandular cells that line the inside of the cervix meet the smooth skin cells that line the outside of the cervix.

V

Vaccine: A method of training the body to recognize disease-causing bacteria or viruses by exposing the immune system to either a portion of the bacteria or virus, or to the whole bacteria or virus that has been made inactive.

Vaginal cancer: A rare cancer of the female pelvic tract that begins in the external area of the reproductive system. It involves cancer of the vaginal tissue.

Vectors: Insects that generally carry infections from animals to humans.

Venereal warts: Body warts in the genital area.

Vertical transmission: Passing of a virus from mother to child.

Vulva: Part of the external female genital system. It connects the vagina to the outside of the body, and includes the inner and outer lips of the vagina, the clitoris (the sensitive tissues between the lips), and the opening of the vagina and its glands.

Vulvar intraepithelia neoplasia (VIN): Precancerous condition also known as dysplasia.

Index